RADEMACHER'S

Universal and Organ Remedies

RADEMACHER'S
Universal and Organ Remedies

(ERFAHRUNGSHEILLEHRE)

ABRIDGED AND TRANSLATED
BY
A. A. RAMSEYER

GYAN

Published by

GYAN

Gyan Publishing House
5, Ansari Road
Daryaganj, New Delhi-110002
Phone: 011-47034999, 9811692060
E-mail: books@gyanbooks.com

Distribution Network
gyanbooks.com
India, USA, Canada, UK, Australia, France

ISBN : 978-81-212-6593-5 (PB)
First Published, 1909

2nd Impression 2022

Printed at: Gyan Press, Delhi.

RADEMACHER'S: Universal and Organ Remedies
Author: A. A. RAMSEYER

RADEMACHER'S
Universal and Organ Remedies

(ERFAHRUNGSHEILLEHRE)

ABRIDGED AND
TRANSLATED BY
A. A. RAMSEYER

"*Prove all things; hold fast that which is good.*"

1909

PREFACE OF THE TRANSLATOR.

What tidings does this little work bring to the medical world? Does it bring forth any new truths, calculated to benefit those who shall read it? The author, Johann Gottfried Rademacher, who was born in 1772, and died in 1850, practiced the medical art in the little town of Goch, in the northwestern part of Germany, during the first half of the XIXth century. He was an observing man, who in 1841 gave in plain, simple language the results of his ripe experience for the advancement of medicine, especially of therapeutics. His work, of which four editions were published, was written in German, appearing in two large volumes of over 800 pages each, from which the following abridged translation has been made.

Rademacher's Erfahrungsheillehre, or empiric medical practice, has at least one merit, it is original. He quotes a few authors, who agree with him, or to whom he may be indebted for his remedies or practice, but the bulk of his work is made up of his own rich fund of experience, with many instructive cases as illustrations. He never assumes a domineering air of superiority, nor does he seek to cover his ignorance with high-sounding, but empty words. In his meek, plain way, he gives out what he knows, for the benefit of his readers, and acknowledges with frankness what he is ignorant of, willing to be taught of others, and ever ready to believe in the good faith of all those who are striving to allay the sufferings of mankind.

His work does not shine with glittering theories or

plausible generalities, but rather with hard facts gleaned upon the practical field of observation in a spirit free of preconceived notions. Yet he must have put up some kind of theory to bind together the sheaves gleaned upon his medical field. Whatever may be the fate of his medical views, whether they must be modified or abandoned, the future will show Rademacher's book as one of the mile stones on the road of medical progress. It has molded, in the past, and in the future cannot fail to mold, the views of those who seek after truth, and who are not satisfied with empty definitions.

We are promised by the great Teacher that by seeking we should find, and that to those who would knock the door should be opened; this is true, no doubt, of medical science, as much as of the gospel. But there are those who are so puffed up by their own learning, impractical though it may be, that they not only refuse to be taught, but would, if possible, make it a criminal offense to teach or to practice any art or science, unless it be in accordance with *their* scientific notions. And yet when it comes to explain scientific facts, theories are being advanced which new discoveries are continually modifying. Those who really know most are more careful in their statements, and do not claim more for their own branch of study than they are warranted to. The superficial mind is always ready to brag of scientific knowledge. Now what is *science?* It is classified knowledge. But who is to do the classifying? Who is so infallible? Let me have rather the following beautiful definition: "Truth is knowledge of things as they are, and as they were, and as they are to come," which definition embraces all things, material and spiritual, in all their evolutions and revolutions, and cannot fail to impress its splendor upon the reflecting mind. What may to-day appear as rank heresy will pass to-morrow as an undisputed truth, while much of the high sounding wisdom of our generation will surely fall and decay in the next. It is not the first time that the weak, despised things of the earth have broken down the mighty and strong ones, and Rademacher's teachings may yet overthrow apparently uncontrovertible axioms.

This translation, although short, is as true and correct as I could make it. I have not always followed the order of pages, but rather the order of thoughts of Rademacher, bringing together what belonged together. Sometimes I had to use words which a literal translation might not warrant, but which the general sense of the sentence required, and transpositions of passages have been necessary to make some passages clear. This book is compact, and, I hope, clear and easily understood. Any chapter, for instance the last one, on "Muscle remedies," will be worth many times its price to the seeker after medical truth.

A. A. RAMSEYER.

Salt Lake City, Utah,
February 8th, 1909.

TABLE OF CONTENTS.

CHAPTER I.

CHAPTER II.

CHAPTER III.

CHAPTER IV.

D. REMEDIES FOR EXTERNAL ORGANS.

XVIII. *Skin remedies.*

XIX. *Muscle remedies.*

UNIVERSAL AND ORGAN REMEDIES.

CHAPTER I.

INTRODUCTION TO RADEMACHER'S ORGAN REMEDIES.

In 1841 appeared in Berlin the first edition of a work which made no little stir in medical circles; in the short space of five years it reached its fourth edition. Its German title* is rather lengthy, but it is generally quoted in short as Rademacher's *Erfahrungsheillehre*, which we may call the empiric medical practice, not of Rademacher alone, but of the old alchemistic physicians, particularly that of Paracelsus. Having practiced that system during 25 years, Rademacher thought it his duty to communicate to the medical world what he knew about it. But in saying system, the reader must not think of this word in the sense of a theory, for, in his preface, the author warns us that he did not pick a so-called theory out of Hohenheim's (Paracelsus) writings, because he held the opinion that there were already too many theories; his (Rademacher's) idea

---

*Rechtfertigung der von den Gelehrten misskannten, verstandes rechten Erfahrungsheillehre der alten scheidekünstigen Geheimärzte, etc., von Johann Gottfried Rademacher.

Justification of the empiric medical practice of the old alchemistic physicians, misjudged by the learned, yet perfectly rational, etc.

was merely to give some plain, rational advice how to make sick people well, not to set up a theory.

Rademacher started practicing medicine in 1795; he left college rather skeptical as to medical theories. Twenty years later, in 1815, when he had had opportunity of gaining a mature judgment in practice, he accidentally came across a remedy which at that time was not found in any pharmacopœia. The remarkable curative properties of this drug (*Natron nitricum*) raised the suspicion that it was perhaps one of the famous remedies of the iatrochemists. His curiosity led him to rummage the writings of *Theophrast von Hohenheim**, and he soon found his supposition confirmed. He decided to thoroughly study Hohenheim; he had not read his works long before he came to this passage, that "the practice must not proceed from the theory, but, on the contrary, the theory must proceed from the practice." This is precisely the standpoint from which we must view all sciences; every newly discovered fact helps us to better understand the theory of matter and forces; from the days of Newton, who discovered the laws of gravitation by observing the fall of an apple, to the days of wireless telegraphy our views in physical sciences have changed, and our theoretical as well as our practical knowledge has been enlarged. Rademacher's object was to make known the excellent virtues of some remedies which he had tried, among them some which the regular school had declared worthless, but which, in his rich experience, he not only found efficacious, but which he declares to be really indispensable. He wrote his book in familiar style, when he was nearly 60 years old.

---

*This is the real name of Paracelsus.

CHAPTER II.

PARACELSUS AND HIS MEDICAL DOCTRINES.

Rademacher seeks to defend Hohenheim against the attacks of his enemies, who had condemned him without reading him. Here are, according to the author, the principal doctrines of that celebrated alchemist:

Disease is something invisible, intangible; the physician must seek its origin outside of the patient, not in his humors, or excretions; he must recognize the *microcosm* (man) in the *macrocosm* (external nature) in other words, he must study natural philosophy; he quotes the following passages: "If ye say, this disease is a disease of *Pulegium*, this one of *Melissa*, that one of *Sabina*, then ye have a sure cure from the name." "A natural and true physician says, this is *morbus terebinthinus*, that is *morbus helleborinus*, etc.; not, that is *Rheuma*, *coryza*, *catarrh*. These names do not proceed from medical knowledge; for similars must be compared with similars in names; from this comparison proceed the cures." "Who knows the number of the plants of nature and of the natural *arcana* (remedies)." "*Contraria a contrariis curantur*, *i. e.*, hot drives cold away, etc., is false, and never was true in medicine; but rather *Arcanum** and disease, these are *Contraria*. The *Arcanum* is the health (principle), and the disease is contrary to the health; these two expel each other, they are the

*The efficacious principle hidden in a remedy.

contraries which drive each other away." "External things alone give us a knowledge of internal ones, otherwise no internal thing can be perceived."

Nearly 300 years before Hahnemann enunciated the law of similars, Hohenheim wrote the same words: "Nullo modo curatur morbus per contraria, sed quodlibet suo simili." And speaking of Tartarus, he says: "Sic similia ad similia addiderunt, et *similia similibus curantur.*" (Vol. I, pg. 398, folio edition of 1603). Yet he must not be understood in exactly the same sense as Hahnemann; the porcelain painter's son was the first one to undertake the gigantic work of collecting the microscopic symptoms of diseases, with their modalities, to apply them to the cure of disease. Paracelsus' idea of the law of similars is a different conception; every organ of the body has its counterpart in nature, for there is an external liver, an external brain, external lungs, etc. By giving the external lungs (Sulphur), so one afflicted with a disease of the lungs, the physiological balance will be reestablished. If the physician understands well the external man, then he can practice medicine, and employ the external man for the internal, and recognize the internal in the external. It thus follows that the prescription must so be made that organ come to organ, the heart to the heart, lung to lung, spleen to spleen. The herbs are the organs; one is the heart, another the spleen, etc. Not that the (external) heart is visible to the eye, but rather it is a spiritual force, and a virtue similar to the heart."

Paracelsus considered natural philosophy, chemistry, and astronomy the foundations of the medical art; not the philosophy of Aristotle, nor the literary baggage of latin and Greek which encumber the curriculum of medical studies, but the study of nature; chemistry was not for him the seeking after the philosopher's stone, but rather the preparation of pure chemical remedies. As for astronomy it was not the astrology of his times; it was what Sydenham one hundred years later called *constitutio epidemica*, something known alone to the observing disciples of Hahnemann and Rademacher. He compares the knowledge obtained from astronomical observation to a letter which has been sent one hundred miles away, and which is understood by its recipient; in the same manner the physician should understand the message of the firmament; this book deceives not, for it is not written on paper. Farther he adds: "If you know not the science of astronomy, then is your work in vain, and the physician is like a fool. Because the remedy does not cure and is of no efficacy, you stand amazed, and exclaim: Well, well! there it stands in the text book, it has cured it there; it must be a plague from God, for I know my art! The only reason is, you are a fool, and know not the concordance of nature."

"Now," writes Rademacher, in explaining the above passages, "I would ask every one who has observed for many years the epidemic constitution and its changes, I will ask every one who has not only treated the sick according to the rules of the school, but who has cured them, whether the efficacy of the remedies is not predicated upon the epidemic constitution, or, as Hohenheim says, upon the heaven? Now an organ remedy soon heals the affected organ in almost every case (with few exceptions), and that evidently. After six months, or a year, or sooner, the same remedy does not accomplish anything in a disease which apparently is the same; but another remedy has again the same rapid and evident efficacy. Even the dose of one and the same remedy is, speaking like Paracelsus, subject to the heaven. We now give the full (*i. e.*, the one dictated by long experience) dose with evident success, and after a while we must reduce the dose to the one-fourth or less in diseases apparently the same. It is then contrary to experience to speak unconditionally of the efficacy of remedies, since this is evidently and mostly predicated upon the heavenly influences of which Paracelsus speaks. As regards the nature of the prevailing diseases and of their changes nothing of general practical applicability can be determined. Should we heap description upon description of such diseases, that would be of as little avail to our posterity as the descriptions given by our predecessors have been to us. We must find out and test ourselves by observation the nature of every prevailing disease."

Hohenheim speaking of such description says: "When that book of the firmament is written on paper, it is only as a shadow on the wall, or as an image in the mirror, which can never give perfect instruction. To be perfectly taught we must see that, the shadow or picture of which appears in the mirror; seing that, we then are not deceived, and need not the mirror, for we see the living thing itself, and from the living thing proceeds our foundation."

This is a really beautiful sentiment, but it does not give us the key to practice. In the following pages*

*The references made to Hahnemann in this chapter are not Rademacher's, but mine. Rademacher, although rejecting the law of similars, speaks well of Hahnemann. (A. A. R.).

I have endeavored to gather the different organ remedies used by Rademacher, with their periods of efficacy. Some day some one may be capable of deducting the therapeutic law of epidemics, when it shall please God to reflect that truth upon his mind.

Kissel, a follower of Rademacher, writing about the changes of *epidemic constitutions*, says:

"This change generally happens in the spring or in the fall; but it is not always at that time. In the year 1848 there was in my district a hepatic affection curable with *Nux vomica*, and which prevailed till May; after that it disappeared, to make room for another affection of the liver which *Carduus marianus* cured, but this lasted till September only. In this month the nature of the hepatic affection was such that *Crocus* was the remedy, and from that time an affection of the same organ appeared which *Chelidonium* cured. Whether these different affections of one and the same organ depend on pathological changes of different portion of this organ, or whether they merely manifest a change in the nature of the disease, I cannot say."*

---

*The late John M. Scudder, too, has recognized this epidemic influence in his medical practice. See "Epidemics" in his Specific diagnosis. For instance, he mentions a period of some 14 months during which *Iron* was almost specific for every disease. (A. A. R.).

CHAPTER III.

UNIVERSAL REMEDIES.

Practical experience taught Rademacher that there are three fundamental affections of the whole organism or system, one of which is cured by cubic saltpetre, another by iron, and the third by copper. Rademacher does not claim that there cannot be more than three, or less than three such affections of the whole organism; in his experience he has found three only. A universal remedy is a remedy which cures an affection not curable by an organ remedy. He has not even unfallible pathognomic symptoms which might characterize each of the three universal diseases, yet in speaking of each remedy, he gives some symptoms which have struck him as generally denoting such an affection, or indicating such a remedy. A remarkable fact that he found out is, that when using universal remedies in acute diseases the fourth day of administration of the remedy is generally the day when improvement sets in. This reminds him of Hippocrates' critical day.

I. **Cubic Saltpeter** (**Natron nitricum**).

In 1814 (in his preface the year 1815 is given), Rademacher was treating a case of acute rheumatism according to the methods of Brocklesly, viz., by bloodletting and with large doses of *Kalium nitricum;* as this salt caused some pain in the stomach, he concluded to try a neutral salt having sodium for base, for he knew that *Natron sulphuricum* acted milder than *Kalium sulphuricum*, and *Natron tartaricum* milder than *Kalium tartaricum*. He gave *Natron nitricum*, which not only did not disturb the digestive tract, but brought about a cure which was bordering on the marvellous. The patient got rid of her rheumatism and of her fever in a few days, without any more bloodletting. The same remedy acted just as well in similar cases; and thinking it might be of benefit in fevers as well as in rheumatism, Rademacher tried it in a case of remittent fever, which had lasted a long while; it cured it in three days. He now tried this salt in different affections, such as angina, pleurisy, scarlet fever, diarrhœa, dysentery, cough, asthma, and many more; the results were excellent, and the cures surprisingly swift. The only fever which would not yield to this universal remedy was the intermittent. With this exception, his practice during eight or nine months was extremely easy and successful, until gastric and hepatic affections and brain fevers appeared which this salt could not cure. So far, he had met with something that was general, common to many affections, and *Natron nitricum* had proved a universal remedy in all these. He was now like an inexperienced rider who exchanges a gentle horse for a stubborn one. He was unhorsed. He had to look for organ remedies, and he found them, too; but these will be taken up later.

The dose of this salt is from one drachm to one ounce for 24 hours. In general two drachms for 24 hours were sufficient; if diarrhœa was present, one and a half drachms were given in a mucilaginous potion or in an emulsion.

Before mentioning the different affections in which he found the cubic saltpetre efficacious, Rademacher warns his readers not to infer from his remarks that it is the best anti-hysteric, antipyretic, etc. He says: "Not so! I know of no anti-remedy against nosological forms. So soon as the same nosological forms, where we saw the most gratifying effects of the saltpetre, are the manifestations of another pathological condition of the whole organism, they cannot be removed any more by saltpetre, but by iron, or copper."

Now follows a partial list of diseases cured with this salt: Hystery, especially in young, plethoric maidens and women. Angina (here along with saltpetre, a digitalis salve externally); in saltpetre angina the tongue is generally coated white. Ophthalmy. Pneumonia and pleurisy, generally with red urine. Cough. Asthma. Epidemics of dysentery in 1819, in 1822, and during the winter of 1832–33. Acute rheumatism. Scarlatina during the summer of 1831. Small-pox in 1817. In both eruptive fevers, the cubic saltpetre mitigated wonderfully the symptoms, and cut the disease short, making the small-pox eruption much less abundant than it would have been if it had been left to nature. The sooner saltpetre was given, *i. e.*, before the fourth day, the lighter were the symptoms; if treated right in the beginning (with saltpetre), these two affections ran a very mild course.

Rademacher found different forms of eruption in one and the same epidemic of scarlatina. Most patients had the smooth variety, a few had small vesicles, and in some rare cases real blisters appeared on the red ground. During an epidemic of small-pox, in 1817, all those who took cubic saltpetre from the beginning of the disease had a very light fever and the eruption appeared in a very mitigated form; one patient had an abundant eruption on the face when he called the doctor in, but, as yet, none on the body, or on the extremities, and the fever was very strong. After taking the cubic saltpetre, the fever abated considerably, and the pocks on the body and the extremities were so few that the disproportion of their number on the face and on the balance of the body was remarkable. It must not be thought that this epidemic was very light; on the contrary, one of the first patients, a fifty year old saddler, was covered from head to foot with the pocks, without a spot of sound skin left; this man died in a very short time after the eruption appeared.

II. Iron (Ferrum).

Qui nescit martem, nescit artem, is an old medical adage—How does iron work in the sick body? "Well," says Rademacher, "I don't know it any more than you do, and we must be satisfied with what our eyes show us. I assure you that I have seen not once or twice, but often enough to be certain of the impossibility of a delusion, patients who were so feeble that they were unable to raise themselves on their bed without help, sit up all alone without any help on the next day after having used two drachms of red (oxide of) iron." Rademacher recommends the tincture of acetate of iron, prepared with sulphate of iron and acetate of lead, as the best and most convenient chalybeate, as it is a mild preparation which does not affect the digestive canal and is very acceptable to the patient even for a considerable length of time.

An important, yet not constant sign of a martial affection (*i. e.*, one curable by iron), is the alkaline reaction of the urine; yet in some martial affections the blue litmus paper turns red. Another probable sign is great debility. A dirty white color of the palate leads to the use of iron, yet it is not a sure sign either. Finally black or purple spots on the skin, especially when they are numerous, also the turning black of a whole limb are pretty certain signs. Rademacher was sometimes led to try iron, or some other universal remedy, after finding the organ remedies useless in this or that affection. Not seldom red eyes, swollen lids, and an increased secretion of the Meibomian glands reveal a martial affection. Sometimes hæmorrhage, generally epistaxis, may lead to the employment of iron. When positive signs indicating iron are not present, it is well to first try the cubic saltpetre.

Rademacher used iron with signal success in the following diseases: Ophthalmia, especially when the lids are swollen; angina; scarlatina; pleurisy; catarrhal consumption; hepatic affections; hystery and hypochondry; amenorrhœa; metrorrhagia; nocturnal pollutions; rheumatism and gout; sciatica; scurvy; morbus hæmorrhagicus maculosus (hæmorrhagic diathesis); dropsy.

In pleurisy iron must be given as long as there is any fever, or the least rest of pulmonary trouble remains, until the patient feels perfectly well.

The tincture of acetate of iron often did wonders in Rademacher's hands in curing bad cases of catarrhal consumption. The dose was one ounce a day. A favorable sign is the clearing of the urine; if it was dark before and it turns to a clear yellow color under the administration of iron, this shows a speedy cure. It looks wonderful to see a patient, who, in the eyes of laymen, seemed doomed, pick up and recover in a short time. But it is not safe to trust to the apparent recovery until the urine turns acid, if it was alkaline before.

Dropsy, like all other diseases, is sometimes a martial affection of the whole organism, prevailing in the kidneys; sometimes it is not a purely martial affection, but rather one combined with an original organ disease. When the urine is alkaline, the indication for iron is pretty clear; yet the urine may be secreted in small quantity and give an acid reaction. It is then well to administer a good renal remedy (solidago or cochineal), by which the urine secretion is augmented, and the urine is then found alkaline. At the same time the physician has the advantage of finding out whether he has to do with an original renal affection or with a universal martial disease; in the first case the renal remedy will cure alone; but if it is a universal disease, the amelioration caused by the renal remedy soon stops, and a universal remedy is indicated. If the urine was alkaline it may take a long time to render it acid again. As long as this is not the case, iron must be given.

Acids, especially mineral acids, are closely related to iron, especially in petechial fever; but the muriate of iron is more speedy in its action, besides patients often object to taking the large quantities of mineral acids necessary for a thorough cure. When Rademacher began his medical practice, iron was reckoned to be injurious in acute diseases, and he himself being under the influence of his time had not much use for it; after learning to appreciate it better, he employed it wherever he used to prescribe the mineral acids. How he happened to find out the virtues of the mineral acids was in this way: Toward the end of the year 1795 he was called to treat a boy, sick with petechial fever. The patient was rational, but had a violent fever, his skin was covered with large black spots, and blood was constantly oozing from his nose. Rademacher prescribed diluted *Sulphuric acid*, which the sick boy drank when he felt thirsty. The bleeding increased, and could not be stopped by external means, so that the patient's life was in great danger. The doctor mixed one ounce of diluted *Sulphuric acid* with just enough water to avoid burning the œsophagus, and bade the boy drink it at once, which he did; but when swallowing it, he let out a cry, and a portion of the acid was thrown up, but the hæmorrhage stopped. He provided the patient with some more acid, with instructions to drink of it as much as possible. The young boy was cured in one-third of the time it took others. Rademacher healed a great many during that epidemic, giving them one-half ounce of concentrated *Sulphuric acid* per diem. The effect was that on the fourth day diarrhœa set in; this was a sign to reduce the dose of acid to one-half, or even to one-quarter ounce, if the diarrhœa was excessive. The black spots disappeared little by little, and so did the fever. This petechial fever differed from ordinary typhoid fevers only by its purple or black spots; there were no red spots. In 1797 Rademacher had occasion to treat typhoid fevers which closely resembled that petechial fever, but *Sulphuric acid* did not do any good this time.

Except in the school of Rademacher, nobody has been using iron systematically in acute fevers, until Schüssler introduced his *Ferrum phosphoricum*, which now by some is recommended as the first remedy in all inflammations. Whether there are or not in nature three general forms of acute disease, curable by saltpetre, iron and copper, it strongly reminds one of the three chronic miasms of Hahnemann, psora, syphilis, and sycosis.

III. Copper (Cuprum).

This remedy, one of, if not the oldest universal remedy of the arcanologists, is not noxious, when employed properly; if it was, the coppersmiths who work in an atmosphere laden with copper oxide, and consequently must take in a lot of it, would be very sickly; but on the contrary, they are healthy. It is true that this remedy is apt to bring about nausea and vomiting; in such cases an addition of cinnamon will moderate or even prevent that. Rademacher used the black oxide, from 1 to 4 grains daily, in doses of ½ or 1 grain, or 1½ to 3 drachms of the acetate tincture daily, with cinnamon water; he claims that when given in proper doses, it acts mildly and agreeably on the human body, and, as it were, increasing life quantitatively; hence its use by the ancient alchemists as a panacea for the prolongation of life. It is useful in acute and in chronic diseases, but universal copper diseases did not come quite so frequently under his observation as martial or saltpetre affections, and their pathognomonic symptoms are much more difficult to elicit than those of the two previous universal affections.

Among the few symptoms which indicate a copper

disease (*i. e.*, an affection curable by copper) may be enumerated an acid urine (which is also the case in saltpetre affections, copper and saltpetre affections having the greatest similarity), a considerable muscular debility, delirium (or at least a weakness of memory, on account of which the correct word cannot be found), and in acute fevers a sudden dyspnœa, which not seldom is the forerunner of great danger, or of death through paralysis of the lungs. The effects of this remedy are so clear, so salutary, and so quick that when it is used as a test remedy it very soon reveals the true condition of the whole organism; the muscular debility disappears within a day, so does the dyspnœa, and the urine turns clear and limpid, if it was brown and muddy; but if it was at first clear and limpid, and then gets darker on giving copper, the physician is on the wrong track. In martial affection, the urine is alkaline in the rule, but sometimes it is acid instead; in such a disease, if copper is administered by mistake, the urine will turn alkaline in two or three days, which is then a sign that iron, the right remedy, must be given now, and copper discontinued.

In enumerating some diseases in which copper proved curative, the reader is warned to remember that it is not recommended as anti-apoplectic, or anti-rheumatic, etc., but as a remedy against all those diseases which are merely different forms of an affection of the whole organism, curable by copper.

With copper Rademacher cured some neuralgias of the head, apoplexy, paralysis, angina and scarlatina, threatening paralysis of the lungs, pleurisy (in January, 1825, he treated several cases of pleurisy and cured them with copper), dropsy, hæmaturia, acute and chronic rheumatism (especially in 1832 and 1833), eczema and herpes, asthma, and worms. Copper does not expel the round worms alive, but it kills them, when given in small doses for a length of time; the black oxide of copper given in 1, 2, 3 or 4 grains a dose four times a day kills the tapeworm, too, head and all, thus differing from turpentine which may only expel some segments, without the head; turpentine has another disadvantage, it makes some people very dizzy, while copper has no antagonistic effect on the body, only on the worms. Copper does not seem to kill thread worms, but expels them alive.

To show its beneficial effects Rademacher cites the case of a young man, formerly employed in a distillery, but now unable to work on account of a humid itching tetter on his arms, trunk and legs, which made his wrists almost immovable; any movement was painful, and he felt an aversion to work and a heaviness in the whole body; he felt weak, was emaciated, his sleep did not refresh him, and was very much dejected by the thought of becoming a burden to others. He was given the tincture of acetate of copper 30 drops six times a day; after taking it for three days, the feeling of lassitude diminished, and instead he soon became aware of a feeling of strength and health, although no difference could be noticed in the appearance of the herpetic eruption; then the itching lessened, the eruption lost its redness and its humidity, a new epidermis was formed, and in three weeks he was entirely well and remained so.

As remedies related or similar to copper in their curative effects, Rademacher mentions wine, brandy and ether. From 1802 to January, 1808, he cured many pleurisies and fevers merely with spirituous drinks, alone or with ether. Wine did not aggravate the delirium, a common symptom of those fevers, but on the contrary by its means the patients regained their reason. The year 1808 was the turning point for a change of diseases and of remedies; after January 17 of that year alcoholic drinks and ether acted injuriously in the diseases treated by Rademacher, and other remedies had to be employed.

Rademacher advises his readers to watch the effects of saltpetre, iron or copper, as their use may lead the physician to find out hidden organ diseases; for instance, a sensation of fullness or pain in the right or the left hypochondrium, following the use of a universal remedy, may denote a hepatic or a splenic affection, calling for the appropriate organ remedy.

CHAPTER IV.

ORGAN REMEDIES.

All through his writings Rademacher gives us plainly to understand that it is by reading Paracelsus that he has gained a real practical insight into the science of medicine. Paracelsus is the most illustrious and the most voluminous alchemical writer, hence we must expect to find in his writings the main points of the practice of the arcanologists. But it is well known that at all times physicians have striven to find remedies that would work on the whole organism. As for organ remedies, such have been found and used from the beginning of the medical art, as may be seen in the works of Dioscorides or Galen. Organ diseases are comparatively easy to find out now (but in Rademacher's days physical diagnosis was in its infancy); yet how few physicians realize the importance of primary (idiopathic) organ diseases! How few know that in many cases these diseases cannot be demonstrated *de visu*, as they reveal themselves only through sympathetic affections of the strangest nature. This cannot be learned from books, the physician must learn it by practical experience. Just as there is in the human body something general upon which the universal remedies act, thus healing if not all, yet most nosological forms (diseases), so does experience teach that there are in nature remedies which cure diseased organs. How that is done is beyond our comprehension, hence it is nonsensical to arrange these remedies according to categories, supposed to hint at the kind of their curative action. Rademacher does not seek the nature of these organ diseases in the body or in the diseased organ itself, but in the outside world; hence he recognizes in every organ as many pathological conditions as there are remedies acting upon that organ, according to his experience. For instance, he knows in the liver a *Celandine*, a *Nux vomica*, a *Carduus Mariæ*, a *Turpentine*, and a *Quassia* disease, but he does not pretend that there cannot be other pathological conditions (diseases) of this organ, and he concedes that physicians may know more hepatic diseases than he does; further there is yet the possibility of an affection of the liver which may be unknown to all, because perhaps its true remedy is not known.

Universal remedies cure independent, original affections of the whole organism only, not sympathetic ones depending from a diseased organ. Again, organ remedies cure primary affections of the organs only, not sympathetic ones (caused by another organ), neither do they cure affections of the whole organism prevailing in some organs.

It is sometimes easy to recognize the primary or idiopathic affection of an organ; but sometimes it is difficult; what we see may be sympathetic symptoms only; these may not direct us to the primarily affected organ which is yet hidden; by repeated observations and trials, and by comparing many cases together, we may arrive at a practical knowledge of the virtues of organ remedies.

A. ABDOMINAL REMEDIES.

I. Remedies acting upon liver and spleen.

SEMEN CARDUI MARIÆ (*Carduus marianus*).

In 1808 or 1810 Rademacher was called to treat a woman suffering abdominal pains, especially severe in the cæcal region; he could not make out whether it was a case of gallstones or of induration of the liver; although he had seen and treated a good many hepatic affections before, all his efforts were of no avail; hectic fever appeared, the face took a muddy, yellowish color, sleep fled, and the emaciation was such that no one doubted but what the patient was dying of consumption. He happened to remember that Stahl praised the seed of the lady's thistle in pectoral inflammations accompanying bilious fevers. The sick woman got a decoction of the seed. The effect was wonderful, for the pains disappeared, and she recovered entirely.

Since that he has often used that remedy, and found out that it is excellent in the sympathetic spitting of blood which not seldom accompanies chronic hepatic and splenic troubles. In acute bilious fevers, with pains in the side, cough and bloody expectoration, it is without a rival. It has cured metrorrhagias depending upon hepatic affections, also dangerous epistaxis depending upon liver or spleen diseases. When sciatica is caused by a primary affection of the liver or of the spleen, this seed cures it. It has relieved many chronic coughs depending upon primary affections of the liver or the spleen. But when treating cough or nosebleed depending upon primary abdominal troubles the physician must be on the look out for acids in the intestinal canal; if such be present they must be neutralized first, else an abdominal remedy can never accomplish what is expected of it. But of this, more later.

No remedy can compare with *Carduus marianus* in gallstone colic. But it is not always easy to recognize this. In general it is well in all cases of abdominal pains, whether they be cramps of the stomach, colic, etc., to notice where the least remnant of pain lingers at the end of the attack; it is here that the primarily affected organ will generally be found.

The efficacy of this seed resides in the integuments, not in the meal. Rademacher used the tincture, 15 to 30 drops a day in a cup of water or milk. But if a sympathetic diarrhœa is accompanying the hepatic or splenic affection, it is a sign that the primary organ affection has greatly increased, and in this case large doses are of no avail; small doses of 4, 3, 2, or even 1 drop four or five times a day alone can help.

MIXTURE OF TURPENTINE AND SULPHURIC ETHER.

This is another remedy which, like *Carduus marianus*, acts beneficially on the liver and on the spleen. Paracelsus claims that this mixture, to-day called Durand's remedy, is beneficial in all indurations.

The mixture is prepared by mixing 16 parts of *Spirit. sulph. æth.* and 1 part of *Ol. tereb.* In treating a patient for gall stones or for induration of the liver, all depends upon the dose. Begin gently with 10, yea, for irritable bodies, with 5 drops in half a cup of water three times a day. Then slowly augment or decrease the dose according as it is borne. After taking the mixture, there often appears a slight pain in the liver, which lasts one or two minutes. Although this symptom is rather desirable, the dose must not be increased until the patient has failed to notice this pain for several days. Watch the urine, too; if it gets darker, and if at the same time the patient complains of a feeling of discomfort in the epigastric region, stop the administration of the mixture and give instead the seed of *Carduus marianus* until that feeling disappears and the urine is clear and yellow. Now start again with the mixture, but in lesser dose as at first, and do not increase the dose very soon. The smallest dose which Rademacher used was ten drops three times a day for a lady of the upper class. She was troubled alternately with chronic diarrhœa, cough with bloody expectoration, her face had a dirty, yellowish color, she had œdematous feet up to the ankles, and emaciation of the body. When the gallstones were troubling her, she suffered a violent pain in the epigastric region which would bring on fainting, spasmodic contraction of the abdominal muscles in the hypogastric region of the right side, vomiting, a decrease of the quantity of urine, muddy, dark urine and an icteric skin. Her body being very irritable, she began with 3 drops and increased them gradually to 10, with such excellent success that she was cured of all her complaints in an incredibly short time. Sixty drops a dose is the largest dose he ever used. But the mixture must be continued for a long time, however quick the relief may have been; half a year is the shortest period of administration.

In regard to obstructions and indurations of liver

and spleen they can sometimes be recognized by touch; they are often accompanied by a lump in the hypochondriac region where the affected organ lies; and such hard lumps which are nothing but contracted fibres of the abdominal muscles covering the affected organ could be mistaken for tumors. These hepatic or splenic obstructions or indurations can be found in two stages; the one when they are at rest, the other when stirred up. Just as there are people who have gallstones without experiencing any trouble from them, so there are people who have partial obstruction of these abdominal organs without being much incommoded thereby; but others may have many symptomatic affections arising therefrom, such as chronic headache, insanity, amblyopy, ophthalmy, chronic cough with or without expectoration, chronic diarrhœa, constipation, hæmatemesis (this, however, mostly with spleen affections), dropsy, almost obstinate epistaxis, and other less important complaints. But when stirred up these obstructions manifest themselves by fever, pains in the side, cough with bloody expectoration, violent pains in the epigastric region and in the back, violent colic, continual vomiting, great anxiety, and sometimes by icterus.

In many cases it is not possible to discover the reason for the change of one stage into the other. A shaking up or some overexertion may bring it about, but while a slight commotion or exertion, even the mere bending or turning of the body, may suffice to bring about a gallstone colic, the commotion must be much greater and of much longer duration in obstructions of the liver or of the spleen to bring about bad effects; among the causes are riding a hard trotter, riding in a wagon without springs on an uneven road, and vomiting, especially that produced by emetics. In the case of gallstones the concussion immediately causes colic, but in obstructions the mischief appears only two or three days later, when the causing factor is apt to be overlooked.

II. Special remedies for the liver.

QUASSIA AND QUASSIA WATER.

In the spring of 1825 Rademacher met with some bilious fevers which had this peculiarity that they showed daily remissions, bordering closely on intermissions; few, but very few, had a light chill at the beginning of the attacks. Many complained of pain in the liver, others had none; most patients had diarrhœa; the pulse differed according to the patients. The urine differed in color, in some it was turbid, in others clear yellow, and in others again yellow as gold. The tongue was not coated. *Quinine* changed the remission into intermission in about three weeks, but that could not be called a cure.

In one case where *Quinine* refused to act, he decided to stop that drug altogether, and gave ½ drachm of extract of *Quassia* merely as a placebo. He was not a little surprised to see the fever disappear when the potion was used up. He tried it on other patients and satisfied himself that he had found the right remedy, but as the *Quassia* aggravated the diarrhœa, or brought it on when it was not already present, he had a spirituous water prepared which perfectly controlled these fevers during a whole year.

But *Quassia* is not only an epidemic remedy, it is an

excellent remedy in dropsy, depending upon an affection of the liver. Against this dropsy diuretics are of little avail, for if they augment the quantity of urine, and make it clear (if it was dark before), this amelioration is not lasting. This *Quassia* dropsy may have as concomitant a chronic diarrhœa, either spontaneous or caused by drastic purgatives. The dose of this quassia water is half a spoonful in water four times a day.

CELANDINE (*Chelidonium*).

During the last months of the summer of 1827, strange fevers appeared which Rademacher, after mature investigation, declared a primary affection of the inner hepatic organ (by which he means that unknown portion of the liver which secretes the bile; in this affection no bile is secreted, hence the stools are white, but the skin is white, too, not yellow, as no bile is secreted, consequently there is none to absorb and to deposit in the skin). This fever began with mixed chill and heat, followed in a day or two by headache, then vertigo; many patients had involuntary sighing (an important sign of hidden abdominal affections); the color of the urine differed very much, being yellowish and turbid in some patients, clear yellow like gold in others, and again of a pale yellow as in healthy people in some others; delirium was not continual in most cases*; the complexion was unchanged in some cases, muddy in others; painless diarrhœa was present

* Rademacher mentions somewhere else that all abdominal affections of primary nature may cause delirium, but none so easily as the *Chelidonium* affection of the liver. He once cured with this drug a case of insanity depending upon such an affection.

as a rule, generally lasting till the patient recovered, the feces being yellow or brown, never gray or white; but what was remarkable in many was that the stools passed unnoticed although the patient was not unconscious, and these involuntary stools appeared on alternate days. During the whole preceding year (1826), another fever depending upon an affection of the pancreas had prevailed which could be cured with *Iodine.* When this remedy failed to act Rademacher knew that another epidemic had replaced the former one.

Quassia was tried, but without success; *Nux vomica* did not help, except in the stage of convalescence, which it shortened very materially. Calomel was given in one case, but it only made it worse. Rademacher, after ransacking his memory happened to think of Celandine, which Ettmüller, an old writer, mentioned as having cured malign pestilential fevers. He got a tincture made (by mixing the juice with enough alcohol until it gets clear and in good condition). This tincture thoroughly cured the prevailing bilious fever in one third of the time it took nature to cure it, and often very imperfectly. If no diarrhœa was present, one drachm of celandine tincture mixed with eight ounces of water and a little gum arabic was the daily dose, of which a spoonful was given every hour. But when diarrhœa was present the dose had to be lessened, and one scruple of tincture mixed with one ounce of gum arabic, three drachms of poppy oil, and eight ounces of water either stopped the diarrhœa, or at least diminished it considerably. The same dose of one scruple had to be given in sympathetic affections of the chest, as larger doses acted injuriously.

To obtain the efficacy of celandine it must be given in small doses, down to one-half scruple doses a day, or even less if necessary. Rademacher met with chronic hepatic affections where he had to come down to 2 or 3 drops of the tincture given four or five times a day. During the summer of 1835 when celandine hepatic diseases were prevailing he treated an adult girl suffering with high fever, violent cough and diarrhœa with tenesmus, and cured her in five days by giving her four times a day a single drop of the tincture diluted in half a cup of water, after getting rid of the very painful tenesmus by an application of Belladonna salve to the anus.

Combination of Muriate of Lime with Celandine Tincture.

For over a year, down to June, 1830, there were prevailing bilious diseases which could be cured with *Nux vomica.* During that month Rademacher was called to a man suffering with what seemed to be the prevailing disease; his fever was moderate with distinct but irregular remissions, the urine, which was of a dark yellow color, pointed to the liver being affected. For the first time the spirit of *Nux vomica*, the epidemic remedy during the past year or two, failed to cure; all the other hepatic remedies known to Rademacher were tried one after the other but in vain. In examining closely the patient's abdomen, Rademacher found on the right side of the stomach a spot which was more sensitive to palpation than the rest of the abdomen. Believing that the stomach was affected as well as the liver, he gave him what he knew to be a good stomach remedy, the Muriate of lime, which, however, did the patient no good. Rademacher now gave the tincture of Celandine along with the Muriate of lime, by way of experiment; this mixture helped at once and the patient got well. Other patients came under his observation; he gave them that mixture (Liq. Calcariæ Muriat. 2 oz.; tinct. Chelidonii, 1 dr.), 15 drops in half a cup of water five times a day, and they were cured, some sooner, some not so speedily; those who had been ailing a long time before taking to bed recovered more slowly than those who got the disease bad from the start and were treated from the beginning of the affection. This is common to all organ diseases. During that summer (of 1830) he cured many people who were affected with the same hepatic diseases, but neither in acute nor in chronic cases did he find again the stomach sensitive to palpation. During the summer of 1834 the same disease reappeared, but, by trying different remedies, he soon found the right one. Yet, with all his perspicacity and good intentions, Rademacher could not describe it more minutely. But he now had one advantage, instead of being led by chance to the right remedy he could try one after the other all those he had learned to know.

NUX VOMICA.

Rademacher used this remedy from 1816 to 1819 with much success in diseases of the liver, which appeared either as jaundice or as bilious fevers; *i. e.*, in the first case the bile was kept back and absorbed, in the other case there was an excessive secretion of bile poured into the intestinal canal, causing fever, colic, vomiting, diarrhœa, etc. The tincture of *Nux vomica* cured both forms, being given in combination with one-half ounce of *Natron carb.* dissolved in eight ounces of water, for twenty-four hours, when the stomach and the intestines were overloaded with acid. *Magnesia*, too, can be used to neutralize that acid.

In the spring of 1829 Rademacher met with some hepatic affections, characterized by dark urine, diarrhœa, after pains in the right side and in the pit of the stomach; no acid was present in the stomach or duodenum. The carbonate of Soda given alone was tried, but did not cure, neither did *Chelidonium;* the tincture of *Nux vomica* did better service, the patients felt better, the urine became clearer, but the diarrhœa increased. He now tried the spirituous water of *Nux vomica* and found the right remedy. This same remedy proved very effective against sympathetic coughs depending upon primary hepatic affections; this cough is not seldom the only symptom which betrays the hepatic disease. Generally this cough is dry, with scant expectoration of a clear mucus, but sometimes the expectoration is abundant, thick and yellow.

Saffron.

In 1836, from the beginning of the year down to June, hepatic diseases were curable by *Carduus Marianus.* When this remedy began to prove inefficacious, Rademacher tried in its place the water of quassia; this indeed cured, but so slowly that it was evident this disease was not a Quassia affection; a patient suffering from acute fever with painful affection of the lungs, cough and bloody expectoration was given Quassia water, but as it proved very distasteful, the patient asked the doctor if it was not possible to give it a different taste. To satisfy him Rademacher added a scruple of Saffron tincture to four ounces of Quassia water, merely to change the color of the potion. But what was his astonishment when the Saffron brought about a speedy cure. This and other cases in which the Saffron tincture was given alone demonstrated the virtues of this drug, which now cured as speedily as the lady's thistle had done in the five preceding months. With this hepatic affection appeared sympathetic bowel complaints, which took the form of a perfect dysentery, viz, fever, abdominal pain, tenesmus, vomiting, and slimy, bloody evacuations without a trace of fæces. This dysenteria hepatica was cured very easily with small doses of Saffron tincture.

III. Spleen Remedies.

Remedies acting upon the spleen are hard to find, writes Rademacher, because spleen affections themselves are difficult to diagnose. As sympathetic symptoms depending upon spleen affections he observed the following: Frequently pain in the stomach, oftentimes a violent, suffocating cough, sometimes abdominal pain, chronic diarrhœa, or constipation somewhat oftener, seldom asthma, often disturbances in the kidneys with a resulting dropsy. Of the dropsies, not depending upon a morbid condition of the whole organism, he ascribes about one-third to the spleen. In females spleen affections affect the womb and the vagina, causing sometimes retention of the menses, sometimes metrorrhagia or fluor albus. Many acute fevers and intermittents are merely sympathetic spleen affections.

Positive signs of a spleen affection are often apparently very insignificant when taken alone. For instance, of what signification may be an occasional fugitive stitch in the left hypochondriac region, felt sometimes before a cough, by a patient suffering of a chronic cough? But in the absence of all signs of a hepatic affection, or of a primary disease of the lungs, such an insignificant symptom is of great importance for the practical physician.

Charcoal.

With this remedy Rademacher has cured quite a few people, but although having used it for a long time he is not quite sure that it is a spleen remedy.

Chronic asthma, with nightly aggravation, may be, like cough, a sympathetic symptom of a spleen affection. Here is an instructive case. "A man affected from his youth with a moist eruption of the whole body, which in his virile age disappeared of itself, leaving, however, an ugly, scaly epidermis, commenced to complain of a tension in the left hypochondriac region; sometimes this sensation degenerated into a slight, dull pain, which soon passed away. It was not on account of this complaint that he sought my help, but on account of a continual shortness of breath. I soon found out that he had felt this sense of fullness in the hypochondriac region much longer than the asthma, hence I judged that he suffered with a spleen affection, which was the more probable since he never before had the least trouble with his lungs. I did not give him Charcoal, but another remedy, of which I shall speak further on, and his ailment lessened visibly. After reaching a certain degree of amelioration he was taken very sick with a bilious fever, which prevailed at that time, and which, in his case, was coupled with a serious sympathetic affection of the lungs. This pulmonary affection did not consist of his previous asthmatic trouble, but of pleuritic pains with cough and bloody expectoration. He recovered, but only so far as to be out of bed the whole day, when his old asthma returned with renewed violence. I again gave him the spleen remedy which had so much lessened his ailment before this last acute disease, but this remedy now did him no good. Asthma and cough remained, and instead of being able to recover from the acute disease by means of nightly rest, the asthma drove him every night from his bed. I now gave him Charcoal; this remedy soon changed the scene. The cough and the asthma decreased, the latter soon disappeared entirely so that the man could visit afoot his friends who lived several miles away."

SQUILL.

Unlike the Charcoal, the Squill is a real, excellent spleen remedy, which Rademacher has often used for those dull pains appearing on the border of the epigastric and of the left hypochondriac region, with an absence of all signs of hepatic affections. He used it with excellent effect, too, in apparent stomach pains which are more or less ameliorated by lying on the left side, and which probably depend upon a primary affection of the spleen.

In 1829 when bilious diseases were prevalent spleen affections appeared oftener than during similar epidemic diseases of the liver, and here the tincture of Squill proved very efficacious, in doses of 15 to 30

4

drops five times a day. But in a case of very painful affection of the spleen the dose had to be reduced to 5 drops five times a day, on account of the diarrhœa which it is apt to cause in certain patients.

Acorn Water (*Spiritus glandium quercus*).

Rademacher was once asked to relieve a joiner of some abdominal pains which had lasted a long time and for which he had sought in vain the help of other physicians; after trying on him all his hepatic and intestinal remedies without any success, Rademacher counseled him to try to get less coarse food, better adapted to his sick abdomen. He lost sight of him for a few years, and then when meeting him learned that he had been cured with the tincture of acorn. The doctor who had since learned something of organ diseases and their remedies asked him to point to the region of the abdomen where the pain last disappeared at the end of an attack. Without hesitating one minute the joiner pointed to the place of the abdomen nearest the left hypochondriac region, thus confirming Rademacher in the opinion that the abdominal pain was the reflex of a spleen affection, the more so since this patient had in vain taken the best intestinal and hepatic remedies. But to make matters sure Rademacher had a tincture of acorn prepared and gave of it a teaspoonful mixed with water five times a day to an old toper who had a painful affection of the spleen and suffered with dropsy, his abdomen being full of water and the legs swollen up to the knees; he thought that if the tincture of acorn had any curative effect on the spleen it would remove, too, the sympathetic kidney disease and the accompanying dropsy. His supposition proved correct. The urine secretion increased visibly; but the patient complained of a tightness of the chest after taking every dose; as this probably was caused by the astringent elements of the acorns, the tincture was distilled. This spirit of acorn did not affect the chest, and the secretion of urine increased still more, the sense of fullness of the oppression in the epigastric region lessened gradually, and against the expectations of all, the doctor not excepted, the old drunkard recovered entirely.

After putting the spirit of acorn to such a hard test, Rademacher tried it in all kinds of spleen affections, some of which were painful, some painless, some easy to diagnose, some merely problematic, and he gained the conviction that he had obtained a remedy second to none in such affections, especially in dropsy depending upon a spleen affection.

Other Spleen Remedies

Are *Galiopsis grandiflora*, *Rubia tinctorum*, *Juniper berries*, *oil of amber*, which is excellent in painful spleen affections, accompanied by hysterical cramps; *Conium maculatum* (hemlock) is very efficacious in some sympathetic coughs depending upon a primary affection of the spleen; this kind of cough is difficult to cure, lung remedies cannot remove it, the seed of Carduus marianus is the only drug that sometimes cures it. Rademacher tried hemlock in cases where the lady's thistle had failed and got excellent results, the patients getting entirely well. Finally tartrate of magnesia (*Magnesia tartarica*) has cured painful spleen diseases which other remedies had failed to remove.

IV. Pancreas remedies.

The signs which point to an affection of the pancreas are extremely uncertain, since they fit more or less morbid conditions of the liver, the spleen, and the cœliac plexus. The diagnosis is rendered still more difficult by the fact that the pancreatic disease causes sometimes very painful sympathetic affections of the stomach, liver, spleen or chest, and thus is apt to lead us astray.

IODINE.

Rademacher learned in the following way to esteem Iodine highly as a pancreatic remedy: he once had to treat a robust farmer who complained of dull pains in the region of the stomach; these pains were not increased after a meal, nor by pressure; as concomitants there was a lack of appetite, considerable emaciation, and great exhaustion; the complexion was dirty, the pulse but little accelerated. This ailment presented many variable phases, sometimes the liver seemed to be affected, sometimes the spleen, now it was the portal system, then it was the cœliac plexus. More than once the deep, dull pain disappeared from the epigastric region and sat in the right, or in the left hypochondrium. Once when it sat in the left side the urine secretion diminished and the abdomen filled with water, and Rademacher, believing this surely was a disease of the spleen with a sympathetic kidney affection, gave him the spirit of acorns, upon which the urine secretion increased, the dropsy disappeared, the pain left the left side and returned to its old place, so that he finally was convinced that it was a disease of the pancreas, an organ for which he did not then know any certain remedy.

It was only a short time before that Iodine had been introduced as a goitre remedy, and Rademacher had had opportunity to use it with great success in hypertrophy of the tonsils and of the salivary glands. The similarity of these organs with the pancreas caused him to try this remedy here, giving 10 drops of the tincture three times a day, upon which recovery followed slowly but gradually, the patient remaining well since.

Late in the summer of 1826 a disease prevailed which was characterized by pain and a disagreeable sensation in the epigastric region; the pain was not severe, some patients did not complain when pressure was made upon the stomach, but others did; in these latter cases the stomach probably was sympathetically affected. The other concomitants of the disease were fever, or absence of fever, discomfort and lassitude, lack of appetite, disturbed sleep; and, if the disease had already lasted a couple of weeks, visible emaciation; a characteristic, constant symptom was the turbid urine (*urina jumentosa*). Until then hepatic diseases, curable by *Quassia*, had been prevalent, and it was the inefficacy of this remedy which called Rademacher's attention to the peculiar character of this disease, which, if it continued its course unchecked, presented other symptoms, such as a dry tongue, diarrhœa, slight delirium, when there was fever; it then extended to the gall ducts, and later abdominal pain was complained of. The doctor arrived at the conclusion that the really affected organ must lay in the midst of the epigastric region, as hepatic and splenic remedies which were used when the liver or the spleen seemed affected did not cure the disease; and this organ must be the pancreas. Hence, he mixed 30 drops of tincture of Iodine with eight ounces of water and one scruple of gum tragacanth, and administered a spoonful of this mixture every hour. The disease disappeared with a surprising swiftness. This affection prevailed for a full year, and then made way for a hepatic disease curable with Celandine.

With the beginning of the year 1835 Rademacher met again with pancreatic affections for which Iodine was the remedy. In this epidemic the turbid urine was the most general symptom, but some patients had a symptomatic affection of the kidneys, which was not the case in 1826. This affection of the kidneys was recognized by the brown urine which did not clear up, although all the other symptoms disappeared. An infusion of golden rod (Solidago) generally removed this trouble in one or two days. This epidemic lasted four months, during which time Rademacher cured many people affected with a chronic cough, depending upon the primary disease of the pancreas. Most patients thinking it was merely a catarrhal cough did not seek medical aid until evident emaciation, lack of appetite, a bad complexion and shortness of breath made them suspicious of a serious ailment. The patients generally complained of a sense of oppression in the region of the stomach; many had, besides, a sensation as if a morsel was sticking in their throat, others complained of difficult deglutition, while nothing abnormal could be discovered by inspection.

Rademacher, being well aware that he has not been able to prove without cavil that Iodine is a pancratic medicine, adds: "In order that my readers may not think that I want to force upon them Iodine as a pancreatic remedy, I will remark that it is the best remedy to stop vomiting, and one of the best remedies to allay severe colicky pains, doing it just as quickly as Opium, from which it might be deducted that it acts just as well upon the cœliac plexus, and that the above described affections it cured so well were merely sympathetic or reflex affections of the cœliac plexus. Who can give us light on this dark subject?"

V. Remedy for the Cœliac plexus.

AMYGDALA AMARA.

In the mid-summer of 1828 a malignant, tedious fever made its appearance; most patients complained of a moderate pain in the middle of the epigastric region; there was a moderate diarrhœa, the urine was clear, almost normal, the tongue clean, the fever was a *continua remittens.* There were no general characteristic symptoms, the only strange thing was that all the patients who had worms passed or vomited them. After trying Iodine in vain, then hepatic and splenic remedies with no more success, Rademacher gave the water of bitter almonds. This was the remedy; the dose was one ounce in twenty-four hours, mixed with eight ounces of some mucilaginous drink, taking one spoonful every hour. Some were cured promptly, others had sympathetic affections of the liver or of the spleen, or of the kidneys, as is the case in all gastric fevers. Of all abdominal diseases which he ever met, none, when left to itself, had such bad sequels as this one; never did he have so many dropsies to treat as after this disease; the dropsy, which sometimes was of hepatic, sometimes of splenic origin, could be cured with Quassia or spirit of acorns. But he did not wait for such complications in his own patients; as soon as he noticed that another organ was sympathetically affected he gave along with the water of bitter almonds the appropriate remedy, Celandine tincture, for instance, for the other organ, thus preventing further complications.

VI. Stomach Remedies.

Rademacher recommends as excellent remedies to stop the vomiting *Bismuthum nitricum*, *Kali aceticum* and *Natron aceticum*. Vomiting may be caused by too much acidity in the stomach; in this case the acid may be neutralized by the *Ammonium carbonate*; two drachms of this salt and one scruple of gum tragacanth are dissolved in eight ounces of water, and the patient is to take a spoonful of this tincture every hour; if the stomach rejects the first or second dose it does not matter, the patient must keep taking this simple potion with which Rademacher has cured many cases of chronic vomiting, even such as had withstood the administration of many remedies. The Carbonic acid which is here set free in the stomach may be the curative agent, since an effervescent wine like Champagne has the same effect.

Iodine, too, is one of the best and surest remedies to arrest vomiting, thirty drops of the tincture being mixed with eight ounces of water, and one scruple of gum tragacanth, and one spoonful administered every hour. It also allays pains in the stomach just as quick as *Opium* or any other narcotic. The muriate of lime (*liquor calcariæ muriaticæ*) Rademacher prizes highly as an excellent stomach remedy, not only in diseases of the stomach characterized by vomiting, but in others where there is present pain, bloatedness after eating, belching of wind, etc.; with it he once cured a man who had had dysentery and who now complained of a strange symptom; every time he ate solid food he became cold as ice and a cold sweat covered his forehead, but he had no pain or sensation of any kind in his stomach.

The vomiting of blood, although serious enough, is not so dangerous as might appear; indeed, Rademacher has seen more than once people who had been complaining for a long time of pain in the left hypochondrium, and who had taken many drugs in vain, get well after vomiting blood; he sometimes went so far as to foretell such of his patients that sooner or later they would vomit blood, warning them not to be afraid if it happened, but that it would relieve the pain. But as it is not possible to know beforehand whether such a hæmorrhage will be beneficial or not, Rademacher recommends the infusion of the seed of *Carduus Marianus* to check it. *Opium* in small doses is a good remedy for that, too, but as it causes fainting in some patients he avoids its use.

VII. Intestinal Remedies.

Most intestinal affections are merely reflexes of primary diseases; liver or spleen affections may cause chronic constipation alternating with chronic diarrhœa, painful or painless cramps, etc. Renal calculus too, may cause the most various sorts of intestinal troubles; so can the plethora of the portal system. What makes matters more difficult is the fact that when chronic diarrhœa or colic depends upon a primary affection of the liver or of the spleen, but little pain may be felt in the hypochondriac regions; and severe (intestinal) colic may be observed without pain in the renal region, and without any strangury.

OIL.

For diarrhœa, even if painful, a simple yet most excellent remedy, especially for children, is a mixture of oil, gum arabic and water, in the proportion of three drachms of oil, one ounce of gum and eight ounces of water. Its good effects extend not only to the bowels but to the biliary ducts, too. Pure oil is better in painful intestinal affections, accompanied with constipation. Mothers would find in oil a better remedy for infantile colic than all the antispasmodic remedies of the drug store. The most serviceable is the oil of poppy, as it is quite mild, and does not turn rancid, if kept in open vessels, simply covered with a piece of linen cloth to keep off the dust and let the air in.

IODINE.

This is a beneficial and quick acting intestinal remedy, which removes abdominal pains (not depending upon acrid matters or impacted fæces) just as *Opium* or other narcotics do; forty drops of the tincture are mixed with eight ounces of water and one scruple of gum tragacanth, and of this the patient takes one spoonful every hour, or every half hour, according to the severity of the pains; thus one dose contains less than three drops.

BURSA PASTORIS.

The shepherd's purse is excellent in chronic diarrhœa, when it is a primary intestinal affection, but is of no use in sympathetic diarrhœa.

MIXTURE OF TINCTURE OF NUX VOMICA AND ASAFŒTIDA.

This is one of the few mixtures wherein great virtues lie hidden. Rademacher once had a patient suffering with excruciating colic which he had failed to relieve; as he was standing by the bed the patient entreated him to do something to allay his pains; Rademacher, to look wise and to appear to be doing something, mixed together two bottles of drugs which happened to be on the table, telling him to take a spoonful every hour during the night. One bottle contained some *Asafœtida*, the other some tincture of *Nux vomica;* the patient had used about one-half of each without benefit. What was the surprise of Rademacher when he visited his patient next morning to find that after taking three doses of the mixture the pain was entirely gone and a sound sleep ensued. Since that time Rademacher saw very few cases of colic which did not yield to this mixture: ℞. Asafœtidæ ʒii, Lutei ovorum q. s., Aquæ ℥viii, Tincture nucis vomicæ ʒiii. M. D. This tincture acts both upon the bowels and upon the liver, and as hepatic colic is the most frequent of all sympathetic colics, this is perhaps the reason why it is so frequently useful.

In a few cases of colic in which the stomach could not retain any medicine, Rademacher used with great advantage a liniment made of soap balsam, or soap spirit, and of caustic ammonium rubbed in the abdomen for half an hour, counting watch in hand. Where this too failed, aromatic air baths, made by covering the belly with a bag filled with curled mint, afforded prompt relief.

Acetate of Zinc.

This salt stops diarrhœa just as well, if not better, than *Opium;* one or one and a half drachms of this salt is dissolved with one ounce of gum arabic in eight ounces of water, and of this potion one spoonful is given every hour.

Mixture of Extract of Catechu and Sal ammoniac.

This is another excellent mixture for diarrhœa depending upon a real idiopathic intestinal affection. The prescription is as follows: ℞. Extracti Catechu ℥i, Salis ammoniaci ℥ss, Gummi arabici ℥i, Aquæ ℥viii M. D. Dose, a spoonful every hour. This mixture is of no efficacy in sympathetic diarrhœa.

Laxatives.

Constipation may cause many disorders, hence laxatives are not to be despised, but constipation as well as diarrhœa may be a reflex of some primary affection which should be found out and cured. In hepatic, splenic and renal affections laxatives, when given in large doses, or for a long time, may change the constipation in a chronic diarrhœa; therefore, prudence must be used, especially in dropsy.

To cure the constipation resulting from atony of the rectum Rademacher recommends clysters of table salt. First ascertain the quantity of salt which, when injected as a solution into the rectum, will cause a passage in about five minutes. Then repeat the injection every day, at the same time gradually reducing the quantity of salt; in this manner the rectum will empty itself, as it regains its normal tonicity. Hypochondry is oft nothing more than atony of the rectum, and can be cured much better with salt water clysters than with drugs. Yet this simple remedy is useful only when the rectum is sluggish.

When there is atony of the whole intestinal canal, as evidenced by the failure of salt water injections, the persistent use of laxatives is very efficacious. Glauber's salt (sulphate of soda), and Rochelle salt (tartrate of potash and soda) are the only ones Rademacher advises to use continuously. With some natures the one agrees better than the other; but the main thing is to have these salts dissolved in sufficient water, one pound of water being the least quantity necessary to dissolve one ounce of salts; more water will not be improper, as the laxative virtue of the salts is increased by the large amount of water. At first the patient may need a large quantity of salts, but he must use less and less daily. For instance he may begin with a cup or a glass full every two hours, and continue to drink till he has a passage, and then stop for the day; in a few days he will soon find out how much he needs to get a daily evacuation. Some use this solution of salts in the morning, some take it at night and get a passage the next morning. By the persevering use of said salts sluggish bowels may regain their normal activity, so that a lesser and lesser quantity of salts will be necessary, until finally the bowels move without them.

When laxatives and clysters fail to relieve the constipation the colon may be at fault, in which case the tincture of colocynth in small doses may bring relief. Rademacher saw two cases where the transverse colon was so distended by an accumulation of fæces that it could be felt as a thick, hard, round roll; the concomitant symptoms were a sensation of fullness in the abdomen, uneasiness, a red, swollen face, increased heat and high fever. After removing a large quantity of hardened fæces with the tincture of colocynth, all the enumerated symptoms disappeared, a proof that the ailment depended merely upon the unnatural accumulation of fæces.

How to Neutralize Gastric and Intestinal Hyperacidity.

There is to be found in the writings of Paracelcus a term which he uses much, but that has been little understood until Rademacher explained what is meant thereby. This is the term *Tartarus*. Says von Hohenheim: "Be diligent and careful, and do not mistake Tartarus for colic, winds or ileus, etc." *Tartarus*, a term borrowed by analogy with the tartar deposited by wines on the sides of barrels or other vessels, means any kind of abnormal excretion or secretion, which acts antagonistically upon the body, and the removal of which is necessary to cure the disease. Renal gravel, stone in the bladder, gallstones, all this is Tartarus; so is excessive acidity of the stomach and bowels. The sympathetic or reflex disorders caused by the presence of gall stones, and enumerated in previous chapters, are not produced by these disagreeable guests alone, for excessive acidity of the digestive tract may cause rheumatism, ophthalmy, amaurosis, insanity, acute inflammation of the throat or of the œsophagus. All these serious troubles may disappear after the use of soda or magnesia, or other neutralizing salts.

Bilious fever or bilious colic in its lightest form depends upon an increased action of the biliary ducts, whereby an excessive amount of acrid bile is generated, filling the stomach and the intestinal canal with acid; spontaneous vomiting, which is not rare in this fever, brings the acid to light, and it is easy to test it with litmus paper. Instead of giving an emetic which may set gallstones in uproar, or seriously disturb the economy, it is safer to neutralize this acid by means of the Carbonate of Soda, or of Ammonia, or with Magnesia. After using three potions of one-half oz. of Natrum carbonicum dissolved in eight oz. of water, with one scruple of Tragacanth to cover the bad taste, the patient will not complain any more of bitter taste, of fullness of the præcordia or of fever. Two drachms of Carbonate of Ammonium are given in the same mixture, to be taken in twenty-four hours. For Magnesia, eight oz. of water and one-half oz. of Magnesia usta are mixed, and form a potion which is easily drunk; but when the potion is allowed to stand over night, the Magnesia lays above the water as a gelatinous mass; in order to mix the Magnesia and the water it is only necessary to break up this mass with a knitting needle, and after shaking it will mix readily with the water. It is astonishing to what degree this acidity may exist in the intestines; sometimes the anus is already sore after two or three liquid stools. The irritation provoked by this acidity may be so great as to cause diarrhœa, which may be stopped by giving alkalies (Carbonate of Soda, of Ammonia). But alkaline salts have this disadvantage: As long as they neutralize the excess of acid contained in the stomach and in the duodenum, they bring a wonderfully quick relief; but when the acidity of these two organs has been neutralized, the soda, for instance, acts locally as pure soda and affects the liver, abnormally diminishing the biliary secretion (Antimony and Opium have this same effect on the biliary ducts); in this case the diarrhœa continues or increases. In such cases crab's eyes are the best remedy; they neutralize the acidity, without affecting the biliary ducts. Such remedies may not only cut short the first stage of a gastric or bilious fever, but the second as well; sometimes, however, it is necessary to add a hepatic to the alkalies, or give oxide of iron with a hepatic, and alkalies when the hepatic affection exists in connection with a martial universal affection.

VIII. Remedies for the Urinary Organs.

KIDNEYS.

The urinary organs may be affected sympathetically by primary diseases of the liver, spleen, etc. An affection of the whole organism may predominate in the kidneys, and call for one of the three universal remedies. Primary affections of the kidneys may cause the following sympathetic or reflex ailments: Unilateral, periodic headache, cough with expectoration, asthmatic attacks, lasting nausea, vomiting, pains in the side and in the bowels, chronic diarrhœa, or chronic constipation, dysury, strangury, red urine, dropsy, pains in the heels or in the soles of the feet, emaciation with accelerated pulse and a pale, dirty complexion and in females metrorrhagia. In many cases of primary kidney disease, urinary disorders proper are absent, the urine may or may not differ from the normal, hence their diagnosis is not always easy.

The alkaline reaction of the urine is frequently met with, and generally indicates iron, as has been mentioned when speaking of the three universal remedies.

The normal reaction of the urine is sour; but this acidity may be excessive, just as is the case with the stomach and the intestines, and this excessive acidity may so disturb the functional activity of the kidneys that the secretion of urine is diminished and dropsy follows. Here are Magnesia, lime water and the alkaline salts, the only permissible diuretics; they diminish the acidity of the urine and restore the normal secretion of urine. Drugs which excite normal kidneys to an increased activy would increase this ailment rather than do good.

The diminished secretion of urine may appear as dropsy from the start, or it may simply cause œdema, accompanied by shortness of breath; again it may cause chronic diarrhœa only. Hence the necessity of measuring the quantity of urine passed during twenty-four hours; by comparing it for several days, it will be easy to know the true condition of things.

Laxatives, such as gamboge, jalap, cream of tartar, and almost all the neutral salts, given either in small or in large quantity, sometimes augment the secretion of urine and may cure dropsy. This method of cure, however, is uncertain, but it is easy, and the kind of dropsy which it relieves is as readily contracted as a coryza, or a cough. Exposure will often bring it about. Rademacher tells of an instructive case: An old clergyman, living in the next town, sent him word to prescribe for a severe abdominal pain. The messenger, when questioned by the doctor, said that the old gentleman was in bed unable to move and continually complaining of pain in the belly; no other precise symptoms could be ascertained, hence the prescription was *Asafœtida* and *Nux vomica.* The next day the messenger returned, requesting the doctor to to visit his patient, who was no better. Rademacher found his belly full of water, the feet swollen up to the calves, and the scrotum œdematous. About ten days before the clergyman had exposed his back to the cold wind, while visiting a sick man in the country, and since returning home his breath became short, his belly stiff, and he had not passed any urine for a long time. A potion of Glauber's salt and powdered jalap taken in copious doses every hour soon restored the old gentleman to health.

Of all the remedies praised as diuretics Rademacher acknowledges only three as such, viz.: *Tartarus boraxatus*, the seed of colocynth, and the diluted tincture of opium. The tartrate of borax has slight laxative virtues; with it Rademacher has cured several dropsies; but when the dropsy depends upon an incurable affection of the liver or of the spleen, the dropsy may disappear, yet the patient will die after getting rid of his water.

To prepare the tincture of colocynth seeds the seeds are cleansed and washed, to remove the bitter dust of the fruit. The largest dose Rademacher used was thirty drops four times a day; often he had to reduce the dose to get diuretic effects. In the case of a female, seventy years old, afflicted with dropsy, he gave fifteen drops four times a day; this did not open her bowels, nor increase the secretion of urine; instead of increasing the dose he decreased it down to seven drops four times a day, diluted in a cup of water; the remedy acted then, and cured the patient.

With diluted Opium (3, 4, at most, 5 drops of Opium tincture mixed with a quart of water, and drunk in twenty-four hours) Rademacher has cured dropsy in several instances. In concentrated form and in such doses as it is given to allay pain, or stop diarrhœa, Opium diminishes the secretion of urine. Many a case of chronic diarrhœa against which massive doses of Opium have proved futile might easily be cured with diluted Opium, since these diarrhœas are caused by a diminished secretion of urine, and disappear as soon as the urine is passed again in normal quantity.

Epidemic Influence in Renal Diseases.

When hepatic (bilious) diseases are prevailing, spleen affections sometimes accompany them, some years being more productive of such anomalies than others. The same is true of renal affections. Rademacher, in all his previous practice, never had so much to do with renal diseases as during the fall of 1829; they were either primary (idiopathic) or followed the prevailing affection of the liver. During the summer the hepatic affection was cured with *Nux vomica*, in the fall it changed and was cured with *Chelidonium*. After the liver had returned to its normal condition, the sense of fullness had disappeared from the precordial region, and the patient felt well again, if the kidneys became affected, the urine which was brown during the hepatic disease, but had become clear again by giving hepatic remedies, either turned brown again or remained clear, but the patients did not get well; the pulse which had become normal, became accelerated again, with the evening came an exacerbation of the fever, and the appetite disappeared. When the renal affection appeared independently of any hepatic disease, some patients complained of fever with pains in the back, some having the pains in the shoulders, some between the shoulders, and some in the loins. By giving the appropriate renal remedy (Cochineal) the disease was cut short and the patient soon cured.

COCHINEAL.

This remedy which still appears in some of the pharmacopœias of the XVIII century, was unknown to the medical world when Rademacher by chance discovered its therapeutic virtues. He had to treat a poor, old female, who, as he thought, was suffering of splenic dropsy; she had a little fluctuation in the abdomen, the legs were swollen up to the knees, the urine was dark and turbid, and she had a lingering fever with cough and expectoration; besides she complained very much of pains in the left hypochondrium. Acorn water was given her and the pain disappeared, but the urine did not increase. To satisfy the woman who thought that the doctor was merely giving her a placebo, Rademacher added some Cochineal to the Acorn water to give it a color, this being the only virtue he knew of the drug. But the Cochineal did more than color the mixture, it entirely cured the dropsy. A second case in which Rademacher had occasion to use it enlightened him still more. A woman of middle age complained of acute fever with stitches in the left side, in the region of the spleen. After using Acorn water the pain left the spleen and settled in the left kidney; a moderate pressure sufficed to make it very severe, and at the same time induced strangury. Cochineal removed this pain in two days; under its further use the fever too left in a few more days, and Rademacher had the satisfaction of learning to know an excellent renal remedy, and was thus prepared to meet the epidemic of renal affections during the fall of 1829, as mentioned above; in that epidemic, whenever the kidneys were affected, Cochineal never failed to cure.

Instead of showing the virtues of this drug by a series of simple cures, Rademacher quotes a few complicated, but instructive ones. The first was that of a woman complaining of very severe pains in the back, and in the abdomen; she passed but little urine, the feet, legs and labia were œdematous, and probably the abdomen was full of water (this Rademacher surmised, as he could not examine her personally); the patient had no rest day or night, on account of strangury, yet the surgeon brought only a little blood with the catheter. A severe metrorrhagia had preceded all this train of disorders. From the fact that renal calculi often cause metrorrhagia, painful disorders of the bladder and of the urethra, and dorsal and abdominal pains as well, Rademacher supposed that renal calculi were causing the mischief in this case; he gave her a potion consisting of one ounce of burnt

Magnesia, two drachms of Cochineal and sixteen ounces of water, directing her to take a spoonful every hour. Her husband reported that after using this potion the dorsal pain was much less, the abdomen not so tense, and the urine secretion restored; the strangury was lessened, she had had one passage; as the urine was still very acid the same potion was repeated, with instructions to take less if the bowels moved two or three times a day. The next report was that the pains had disappeared, the abdomen was not swollen any more, and the feet œdematous only as far as the ankles; the urine being still acid, in spite of the Magnesia, the potion was ordered repeated. The following report was that all was now in order; the urine was still a little acid. The prescription was now two ounces of milk sugar with two drachms of Cochineal in powder form, of which she was to take a spoonful five times a day. The patient recovered entirely.

Another interesting case is that of a pregnant woman, who was attacked with asthma a week before calling for Rademacher. The pulse was quick and full, the dyspnœa great, augmenting toward the evening, so that for a week she had not been able to lay down or sleep; the face was red and bloated, the tongue had a thick, white coat, the urine was abundant; and she had had no passage for three days. The prescription was one-half ounce of burnt magnesia, two drachms of cubic saltpeter and eight ounces of water, of which potion she was to take a spoonful every hour. After using two such potions many symptoms were removed, but the pulse had the same frequency, the asthma, although somewhat attenuated, was still present, and hindered the sleep, and the urine still showed much acidity. Rademacher suspected that the asthma was kept up by a renal affection, therefore the third prescription consisted of one-half ounce of magnesia, one drachm of Cochineal and eight ounces of water, one spoonful every hour; upon which the asthma diminished, a copious expectoration set in and the sleep returned. After repeating this prescription, and then giving the Cochineal in powder, one ounce of sugar of milk with one drachm of Cochineal, one teaspoonful of this mixture five times a day, her condition ameliorated still further from day to day, and the appetite returned, but the pulse remained frequent, the cough and the expectoration did not cease, the urine lessened in quantity, turning red and turbid. Now the patient was given half an ounce of Golden Rod, covered with five cups of boiling water, to be used in twenty-four hours; after using the first half ounce the urine lost its turbidity, after the second portion it lost its red color, after the third it increased in quantity, and under the continued use of the same remedy the patient recovered all her health. The Golden Rod was administered perhaps longer than needful, to make the cure certain.

A third case that illustrates well the therapeutic acumen of Rademacher is as follows: On the 26th of October, 1829, he was called to take in hand a farmer's wife whom another physician had treated for metrorrhagia; he had stopped the bleeding with sour drops, and wound up with a purgative, whereupon a extremely dangerous diarrhœa had set in which could not be stopped, five stools in an hour being the average; she was so weak that she could not sit up, and the excrements were passed into the bed; the abdomen was very painful, the pulse small and frequent, the urine was acid and copious, in proportion to the diarrhœa; she complained of constant nausea and eructations, alternating with vomiting of tasteless mucus; she had been in this bad plight for two days when Rademacher was called. By using some intestinal remedies the diarrhœa was lessened about two thirds, but in spite of his questions and physical investigations, Rademacher could not make out what organ was primarily affected; was the liver affected or was it the kidneys? He decided to give Cochineal for the following reasons: The urine was not copious, of itself, yet more so than it should have been, considering the excessive diarrhœa; again, the nausea was constant and unchanged, although the diarrhœa had considerably abated; now this pointed to a renal more than to a hepatic affection; for, which affection causes a more lasting nausea than kidney disease? Hence his prescription was *Sacchari lactis*, 2 oz.; *Coccinellæ*, 2 dr.; a teaspoonful every two hours. The next day the diarrhœa had stopped, and the whole condition was much better, although the pulse was still frequent. The same remedy was repeated in smaller dose, the belly lost its sensitiveness, the nausea and eructations ceased, the wind passed freely, and constipation set in, so that injections had to be resorted to. Rademacher did not see her from the 5th to the 19th of November, when he was called again, as the urine had turned yellow and turbid, and copious night sweats had made their appearance. The liver was affected, it was very sensitive to pressure, and the abdominal muscles were stiff and contracted where they touch the liver. Celandine tincture was now used, and recovery soon followed. Celandine was the epidemic remedy for hepatic affections that fall.

Here is an interesting case of neuralgia cured with Cochineal: A middle aged woman complained of moderate fever, accompanied by a periodic neuralgia, extending from the right cheek bone over the right side of the frontal bone up to the right frontal eminence, and affecting the right eye ball; the urine was very copious, of normal yellow color and acid. The patient complained of a peculiar sensation of coldness, extending from the upper part of the shoulder blades down to the small of the back, and this sensation of coldness, which was entirely subjective, increased during the exacerbation. Such one-sided neuralgic headaches were not rare in 1829, and had generally been removed with the water of *Nux vomica*, which was the epidemic remedy for the then prevailing hepatic disease, but in this case *Nux vomica* did no good. Rademacher's attention being directed to the copious urine, he tried the Cochineal as powder, and cured the woman. But he warns his readers against considering Cochineal as a specific for prosopalgy; he used it in another similar case, but it only aggravated the evil, which yielded to Celandine, which was then the epidemic remedy for hepatic diseases. Prosopalgy often depends upon a primary affection of an abdominal organ, which must be cured according to the prevailing epidemic influence. He further suggests the trial of Cochineal in diabetes, having seen it bring the increased secretion of urine back to its normal quantity.

Golden Rod (*Solidago virga aurea*).

This is an old and tried nephritic; Ettmüller praises it very much. It would be just as silly to call it a diuretic as to call *Nux vomica* or Celandine a cholagogue. It is an appropriate remedy for the kidneys, bringing them to their normal condition when they are affected. It has proved excellent in those acute gastric fevers when the urine became dark and turbid, although the patient had been getting better, but the amelioration was at a standstill, or was not progressing fast enough. Rademacher explains this by supposing that the original disease has left the abdominal organ and taken its seat in the kidneys. Metastases are not very rare. Hence, it is well in acute and in chronic diseases to keep a watch on the kidneys.

Rademacher uses the infusion of the Golden Rod; half an ounce of the plant is covered with five cups of water and allowed to steep for half an hour; the infusion is then poured off and used during 24 hours.

Gravel and Renal Stones.

There are no characteristic symptoms to recognize gravel and renal calculi, which may sometimes cause pains in the loins or strangury; but as in other renal affections many strange symptoms may be caused, such as cough, cramps of the chest, pains in the side, continuous nausea, chronic diarrhœa or constipation, fetid smelling urine, pains in the heels and soles of feet, painful affections of the liver and of the spleen, jaundice, enlargement of the spleen, abdominal pains, asthmatic attacks, onesided headache, paralysis of the lower extremities, sciatica, dropsy, consumption, dyspepsia, great acidity of the stomach and of the bowels, chronic vomiting, hysteria and metrorrhagia. These are some of the complaints caused by gravel, or by renal stones when disturbed but slightly; when they are in uproar there may be severe colic with vomiting, and in patients disposed to cramps, all kinds of cramps which are given all sorts of Latin and Greek names. When these renal guests are not disturbed the patient is not at all troubled by them.

Magnesia or lime water are excellent remedies for renal calculi; burned Magnesia given conjointly with Cochineal is exceedingly useful for gravel, not only allaying the symptoms present, but at the same time promoting the discharge of sand; warm fomentations on the renal region (bran mixed with warm water) are a palliative not to be despised. These remedies must not be considered as lithontriptics; at least, if they do dissolve the renal stones their action would appear to be exceedingly slow; but they allay the attacks, and that is much gained. All those who have calculi must avoid commotions, and live moderately; if they eat too much, or eat something that causes flatulence, the renal stones are soon in motion. Yet it is remarkable that renal, like biliary calculi, sometimes stand much shaking and motion of the body, without causing any trouble, while at other times a single false step, or a single motion of the body can bring about the worst attack of renal colic. Rademacher saw twice the tincture of *Nux vomica*, given for some hepatic affection, cause renal colic in patients affected with nephritic calculi.

Kidneys which harbor stones, harbor gravel too, as a rule, and as the gravel leaves its hiding place from time to time, in the form of single grains or as fine sand, its detection is easy. In all the chronic diseases which may be thought to depend upon the presence of gravel the urine must be examined daily for two or three weeks in the following manner: Preserve the urine in a covered vesel, to prevent sand falling into it; gently pour the upper part of the urine off the vessel, so as to keep the gravel in the lower portion; empty now this last portion in a glazed plate, and after waiting a few minutes for the gravel to settle down, rub the convex side of a metallic spoon over the bottom of the plate; if the urine contains gravel, this will be distinctly felt, and if the gravel is coarse it will make a grating noise which can be heard several feet away.

It does not follow because the urine is clear that it does not contain gravel. Rademacher oftener found gravel in clear than in turbid or dark urine; neither should age deceive; young women suffering with hysterical symptoms may pass gravel just like older people.

Patients who are known to have renal calculi or gravel must be cautioned, after being relieved of the acute symptoms, that sooner or later the complaint is liable to reappear.

Shepherd's Purse (*Herba, or Thlaspi bursæ pastoris*).

Quite accidentally Rademacher discovered the virtues of the bursa pastoris in gravel affections. A woman whom he had eight or ten years before freed of much gravel, by means of Magnesia and Cochineal, now sought his help as she was in a precarious condition; the abdomen was full of water, the legs œdematous and the urine red, with a bloody sediment. He gave her thirty drops of the tincture of *Herba bursæ pastoris*, five times a day, intending to stop the renal hemorrhage, but to his great astonishment she passed such a copious amount of gravel as he had never seen; he directed her to continue the remedy, and had the satisfaction of seeing not only the gravel cleared away but the dropsy as well. Since that he employed this remedy in so many cases that he recommends it as worthy of all confidence. He tried it once as *reagens medicum* in a woman, 30 years old, who was complaining of a variety of disorders, which made him suspicious of gravel; he failed, however, to discover any by his usual method of investigation; but after using the tincture of Shepherd's purse she passed a lot of fine gravel, which his old eyes could not see, but which grated very distinctly under a metallic spoon.

IX. Uterine Remedies.

There is a close sympathy between the womb and the abdominal organs, and metrorrhagia often is but the reflex of an idiopathic disease of the liver, of the spleen, or of the kidneys. A decoction of *Carduus marianus* will stop a severe hæmorrhage which may have resisted the use of all possible astringents, because it merely was arising from an affection of the liver, or of the spleen. The same is true of Cochineal, and with it Rademacher cured a metrorrhagia depending upon a renal affection.

For painful menstruation he recommends a mixture of equal parts of tinctures of *Nux vomica* and of *Cas-*

toreum, thirty drops five times a day, given a couple of days before and continued during the entire menstrual period; by repeating this remedy at each period the complaint will at length be cured.

Young plethoric girls sometimes have many disorders at the time of puberty. Rademacher often found the nitrate of soda the most effective remedy against these ailments.

When young women are sickly, and at the same time complain of suppressed menses, unexperienced physicians apt to attribute this sickly condition to the absence of menstruation, give iron to bring its return; forgetting that the sickness may be the cause, not the result of the amenorrhœa; in such cases iron may do more harm than good. The organ that is diseased must first be found out and cured, then the menstruation will regulate itself.

The impregnated womb sometimes predisposes a woman to excessive acidity of the stomach and bowels, but the accompanying train of symptoms, such as heartburn, belching, gnawing sensation in the stomach, etc., often disappear after confinement, yet the whole intestinal canal of the mother being still full of acidity, the new born suffers of diarrhœa with green excrements, colic, etc. Now instead of physicking this frail bit of humanity, let its mother partake freely of soda to neutralize her own acidity. It is always well to remember that the milk of mothers is often a fruitful source of the colics and cramps of sucklings; then give the little ones a little sweet oil or a solution of gum tragacanth (which last drug does not turn sour), and give the mother half an ounce of soda daily. Do not give Magnesia either to the mother or her suckling, as it forms a laxative salt with the intestinal acid; sucklings, if they are weak, cannot well stand its inimical effects. It would be best to give the mother some carbonate of soda or of ammonia, as these do not form laxative salts with the intestinal acid.

Very severe metrorrhagia is apt to be caused by miscarriage in the first months of pregnancy, which naturally ceases when the fœtus and the afterbirth are expelled. But the most severe cases of metrorrhagia are those caused by a portion of the afterbirth remaining in the womb. Of all remedies the solution of iron chloride (*liquor stypticus*) is the best to stop this hæmorrhage; complete cessation, however, can only be expected when every vestige of afterbirth has been expelled, but it seems that the iron promotes this expulsion.

Cubic saltpetre is very useful for false pains during labor. It is better than *Opium.* Saltpetre is excellent too in milk fever, but the physician must remember that a chronic disease of some abdominal organ which may have been acquired during pregnancy, but remained in abeyance, is often intensified by the milkfever. In such case cubic saltpetre may do very little good. The organ that is really affected must be cured.

Afterpains, like dysmenorrhœa, can be removed by a mixture of *Nux vomica* and *Castoreum* tinctures.

In real, primary affections of the womb, when after confinement this organ is painful and fever is present, Borax is the best remedy. Rademacher values Borax as an excellent uterine remedy worthy of all confidence.

Lying-in women offer a peculiarity which physicians

will do well to bear in mind, viz., their body is in an irritable condition, so that as a rule they must be given much smaller doses of remedies than other patients would require, be they male or female; one-half or even one-fourth of the usual dose is all they need, otherwise the drug makes them worse instead of better. This is true even of remedies which have no inimical effect on the body; those which are inimical should not be employed at all for such patients. Great prudence must be used and all harsh measures or remedies avoided.

The physician must pay great attention to the prevailing epidemic influence, if he will cure lying-in-women suffering with fevers. The same is true in regard to married women; it is not always easy to decide whether a young married woman is suffering with some prevailing epidemic or whether it is the sickness of pregnancy. Here is a case to the point. In the beginning of 1830, when hepatic affections, curable with *Nux vomica* water were prevailing, Rademacher was called to a newly married woman, who for the last ten days complained of incessant vomiting; the pulse seemed to be regular, the tongue was but slightly coated, there was no fullness or oppression in the præcordia, the urine was turbid, the sleep disturbed and not refreshing, the menstruation, which was due two weeks before, had not made its appearance. Was she pregnant or was she under the influence of the prevailing hepatic affection, which sometimes presented vomiting, and almost always fullness and oppression in the præcordia? With his best stomach remedy, the muriate of lime, Rademacher tried to stop the vomiting, but without success, although it was lessened some; the *Nux vomica* water, which was the epidemic remedy, cured this patient. He warns the unexperienced physician against allowing himself to be deceived by the non-appearance of the monthly, the enlargement of the belly, which may simulate pregnancy. After waiting for five or six months, the patient now has a yellow, or dirty complexion, a lingering fever, pains in the præcordia, and the abdomen filled with water, and it is not an easy work to rid her of her dropsy.

A salve made of one part of extract of *Digitalis* and eight parts of wax ointment and applied several times a day on inflamed breasts has been used with good success by Rademacher for the resolution of enlarged portions of the milk glands; saltpetre was administered at the same time, on account of the high fever.

Rest as a Condition of Cure in Abdominal Affections.

Affections of abdominal organs, whether they be obstructions, enlargements, tumors, etc., present themselves under two different stages, that of quiet and that of excitement; physical exertion, commotion of the body, and mental shocks often bring the affected organ from the quiet stage into to that of turmoil, but it may be two or three days before the effects of such shocks manifest themselves through sympathetic disorders of other organs. *Carduus marianus* is an excellent remedy to allay these reflex disorders. The attention of the reader has been called to this before. But another very important item is that rest of body and of mind is a necessary condition of cure. Sometimes a patient is found who does not feel the necessity of lying in bed, but moves around in or out of his home, and the physician wonders why a remedy which has rapidly cured worse cases refuses its benign effects in such apparently milder cases. Let such patients remain quiet, and it will not be long before his disease too will be amenable to the proper remedy. Rest of body and of mind is an important factor in the cure of diseases.

B. THORACIC REMEDIES.

X. Cardiac Remedies.

Affections of some abdominal organ may cause an irregular intermittent pulse. Rademacher saw a case where gall stones caused such a dyspnœa and an irregular pulse that he was in doubt whether it was not a case of hydrothorax, but *Carduus marianus* soon quieted the gall stones.

The sympathetic disorders caused by organic heart diseases are: Hydrothorax and dropsy; spitting of blood; convulsive constriction of the larynx causing suffocation; hepatic affections with increased or decreased biliary secretion; gastric affections, in the form of fullness in the præcordia, or of constant nausea; renal affections with diminished urine secretion; transitory paralysis, or troubles of the brain functions.

Digitalis is the best cardiac remedy, when given in proper doses. Rademacher prescribed from ten to fifteen grains of the herb steeped in eight or twelve ounces of water and boiled down to half its bulk; the patient is directed to take a spoonful of this decoct four times a day, so that the potion is used up in two or three days. Generally one potion is sufficient to quiet the heart and to remove the sympathetic disorders, such as dyspnœa, oppression in the præcordia; so soon as these disappear, the use of the medicine is left off, although some may yet remain. The *Digitalis* removes the water from the chest by way of the kidneys. True it will not repair structural changes of the heart, and the patients finally die of hydrothorax, but this drug may be used time and time again to rid the chest of its water, and the life of the patient may thus be prolonged.

The sympathetic affections depending upon cardiac lesions are generally removed by *Digitalis;* but it may happen that such a reflex affection has become a real (primary) disease; in such a case the appropriate remedy for that organ must be given. For instance, a man laboring under a heart disease, suffered with sympathetic oppression in the præcordia, especially in the right hypochondrium, which *Digitalis* failed to remove; but after giving him *Quassia* water the uneasiness in the præcordia disappeared, and the urinary secretion became normal. In another case of reflex biliary disorder, the bitter taste and the other symptoms of gastric acidity soon disappeared by giving *Magnesia*, in such doses as to produce three or four stools a day; afterward the *Digitalis* exerted its wonted effects.

It is absolutely necessary to notice the condition of other organs; for if any have been affected previously, and are affected at the same time as the heart, it is sometimes impossible to succeed with *Digitalis* alone, because one organ reacts upon the other, whereby the cardiac affection is exceedingly increased. By treating the organ which was first affected, the cardiac affection is very much lessened, or the way is opened for the exhibition of *Digitalis*, which then does not fail to show its diuretic virtues; for instance, after giving *Sulphur* internally and applying leeches to the anus, in disorders of the portal system. This and other abdominal organs must especially be looked after by the physician.

It is well also to pay attention to the general condition of the patient and see whether a universal remedy is not indicated. For instance the patient may feel very uneasy, the urine may be dark red and acid, the nights sleepless, and the heart's action very tumultuous; after giving cubic saltpetre for several days this condition may be very materially ameliorated, and *Digitalis* may display its excellent virtues. The same may be true of iron, which alone or with *Digitalis* may restore the normal urine secretion in heart diseases.

Severe physical exertions, running, lifting heavy loads, or a fall are apt to induce structural lesions of the heart. Even dynamic (functional) affections of the heart after being cured require a careful avoidance of emotions and such exertions as dancing, jumping, etc., which fatigue or excite the heart.

An intermittent pulse may be caused by abdominal affections as well as by heart diseases; and again some cardiac lesions are accompanied by a quick, although rhythmally normal pulse, so that when such a pulse is met in doubtful cases it is well to auscult the heart. Some people are apt to get an intermittent pulse from trivial ailments. Rademacher once met with an epidemic fever, in which acids, especially *Sulphuric acid*, given in moderate doses caused an intermittent pulse;

and he observed the same in regard to the bark and the extract of Catechu. He once cured a heart affection, which, remarkably enough, was characterized by a perfectly normal pulse. The patient complained of pain in the region of the spleen, lack of appetite, debility, etc., for which he was given two ounces of the powder of *Carduus marianus*, to find out whether this was perhaps a spleen affection. After using this powder (a teaspoonful four times a day), the pain in the side disappeared; but in its stead he now complained of a disagreable pulsation in the stomach, while the lack of appetite and the debility remained the same. Rademacher placing his hand on the patient's stomach discovered an indistinct beating, synchronous with the pulse, and moving his hand over to the heart region felt the heart's excessive pulsations as distinctly as if he had held the beating heart in his hand, yet in regard to frequency and regularity, the beat was perfectly normal. He gave him now a weak decoction of *Digitalis*, and two weeks later when the patient returned the excessive strong beating of the heart had disappeared, the heart beat was normal in every particular, and all the patient's complaints had been removed. As a matter of precaution he was given another infusion of *Digitalis* (one scruple of herb in eight ounces of water, boiled down to four ounces), of which he was to take one spoonful twice a day.

In 1837 Rademacher used the root of *artemisia* with great advantage in three cases of heart affection, after giving *Digitalis* without much benefit. Another case where *Digitalis* proved inefficacious too, was much benefited by crushed fresh melissa laid on the tumultuous heart. In 1839 he cured or greatly benefitted two cases of palpitation of the heart by means of Sal ammoniac (a heaped teaspoonful five times a day). This last remedy is one which has been used by ancient physicians for similar affections.

XI. Lung Remedies.

SAL AMMONIAC.

This remedy which exerts upon the system a similar action to the saltpetre, although weaker, is the best to check the excessive secretion of mucus from the lungs, It is excellent too in suppuration of these organs. Rademacher gives two drachms of Salmiac in twenty-four hours, dissolved in four ounces of water; to cover the salty taste ten grains of gum tragacanth are added, and ten grains of extract of henbane; the patient is directed to take two spoonfuls eight times a day.

This remedy is excellent to heal up abscesses of the lungs, yet Rademacher does not wish to be understood as if Salmiac could cure every such abscess. He is inclined to believe that it is efficacious when the abscess is not too large; but having seen consumption healed by some very simple remedies, such as a little opium, or henbane, or a milk diet, and in one case the drinking of cucumber juice, he is rather skeptical in regard to attributing to drugs the cure of fistulous lung abscesses. At any rate he warns physicians who might witness the healing of one or possibly two abscesses, not to brag of their skill; other abscessess may yet break out and carry the patient to his grave in very short time.

A combination of *Digitalis* and *Opium* is sometimes

of great value to stop the cough and catarrh which threaten to turn to consumption. First a decoction of *Digitalis* is given the patient until his system is visibly affected by the drug, then *Opium* in very moderate doses is administered, whereupon the cough, the expectoration and the fever disappear and the patient recovers.

Golden Sulphide of Antimony.

(*Sulphur auratum antimonii*).

The golden sulphide of antimony is a remedy of exceeding great value in lung affections. In 1800 or 1801 Rademacher was asked to prescribe for a woman who was suffering with a severe cough; after using *Opium*, quicksilver, *Digitalis* and other heroic remedies she only got worse and had to keep to bed. At the end of his wit (he was then a young practitioner), he prescribed a powder of ten grains of Rad. Inulæ, ten grains of Iris florent, and one grain of golden sulphide of antimony. The patient, who was almost consumptive, recovered entirely, and from that time on Rademacher often used this drug, with pure sugar of milk, in affections of the lungs with cough, whether accompanied or not with fever, with or without pains or dyspnœa. The dose is from four to ten grains in twenty-four hours, one grain four times a day being the normal dose.

"It would be a great error, writes Rademacher, to believe that the golden sulphide of antimony must cure all kinds of cough known under the name of catarrhal cough. It is no such wonderful remedy, and is curative only of one peculiar affection of the lungs, differing from other lung affections which are under the curative influence of Salmiac, or of other lung remedies; this antimonial lung affection, like the acute prevailing fevers, depends in many things upon atmospheric causes which are entirely unknown to us. Then it would be a grave error to believe that because the golden sulphide of antimony is a good lung remedy that it must cure, if not all, at least most all so-called catarrhal coughs. This may be the case for years. I have used it, I don't know how long, with excellent success, and used it so often that I might easily have gotten into the notion that it must always go that way. But the truth is that things do not always go that way; other years come too, and many of them following each other, when this remedy is of no use against the catarrhal cough (according to name); partly because these are false coughs, which merely have the form of a catarrhal cough, but are in reality sympathetic lung affections depending upon a more or less obscure primary affection of some abdominal organ, or of the brain, or of the spine; partly because they are affections of the whole organism, manifesting themselves in the lungs under the form of coughs, but which are under the curative power of the one or the other universal remedies. In spite of the prevalence of so-called catarrhal coughs, I have had but little use for the golden sulphide of antimony for several years, because the supposed colds with their coughs were not primary lung affections, but idiopathic liver affections, and previous to this period of gastric disorders were mostly brain and spine affections. 'Tis true, a few cases sometimes slip in which require the golden sulphide of antimony; but they are so few that it is hardly worth to speak of them. For instance, writing this in the beginning of August, 1830, I have during the last seven months given this remedy but twice with benefit, although the presumed catarrhs for which medical help was sought were extraordinary frequent. All other coughs were reflex affections depending upon a hepatic disease, and were cured with nux vomica water. To see in one and the same disease (nosological form) a good remedy refuse its often and long tried efficacy is something well calculated to delude. If there is anything which can not only make the young physician doubt the theories of his master, but make him a real skeptic, it is this fact. Hence, as practical writer I hold it my duty to represent things as they are really found in nature. From such deception easily proceed skepticism, contempt of all methodical art, reviling of the heretical teacher, indifference in the treatment of the sick, medical juggling, and other bad faults which make the medical profession contemptible in the eyes of the people."

The golden sulphide of antimony not only cures a cold with its cough, but it may prevent consumption, provided the epidemic influence corresponds to this remedy.

Extract of Tobacco.

Rademacher learned from Ernest Stahl the use of this extract as lung remedy; but instead of preparing it from the *nicotiana tabacum*, which has a bad smell, he gets it from the *nicotiana rustica*, which has no such smell, provided the leaves are pressed and the juice boiled down at once; if the leaves, after being plucked, remain but 24 hours unpressed, a change goes on which gives the extract a taste similar to that of the smoking tobacco. It is given in doses varying from ½ to 2 grains, or from 2 to 8 grains in 24 hours.

This is one of the best remedies there is for coughs caused by real, primary lung affections; it is excellent also for bleeding lungs or bloody expectoration, if it is an idiopathic, not a reflex affection; and it will prevent consumption just as well as the golden sulphide of antimony, provided the affection is under the power of tobacco.

Blood spitting and hemorrhage from the lungs are considered very serious things. But, although these may be symptoms of incurable diseases of the lungs or of other organs, it does not follow that when plethoric, well fed, otherwise healthy people have a hemorrhage from the lungs that it should be any more serious than nose-bleed.

The extract of tobacco is to the pure, idiopathic hemorrhages of the lungs what the seed of carduus marianus is the reflex hemorrhages, depending upon some abdominal disease. But it is plain that in all idiopathic lung hemorrhages the condition of the whole organism murt be considered. It is sometimes affected, especially in young people, and generally is, although not necessarily, under the curative power of the cubic saltpetre. Then it is proper to give the extract of tobacco with the saltpetre. Again there are hemorrhages of the lungs which like those of the nose, or of the womb, or of the kidneys, are manifestations of a martial disease. Here tobacco extract would be out of place. Furthermore, idiopathic lung affections can affect abdominal organs, and vice versa, and these affections, if not checked and removed early, aggravate each other.

Sulphuric Ether.

This drug given in frequent doses, 2 ounces being administered in 24 hours, is a potent remedy against threatening lung paralysis, which suddenly befalls apparently healthy people, and seems to be to the lungs what apoplexy is to the brain. A two days' use of the ether will remove the dyspnea; the remedy must then be given less frequently, and in smaller doses.

Sugar of Lead.

Lead has been vaunted as an *anti-phthisicum.* Rademacher, although not endorsing this claim, recommends it in conjunction with iron in certain consumptions, adding that it is a universal remedy, as well as iron, and that it acts like iron, but displays some antagonistic effects upon the alimentary canal. Most of those to whom he gave the acetate of lead sooner or later, sometimes two weeks after ceasing taking it, got a moderate diarrhœa, which lasted several days, and was generally painless: Being of the opinion that it was an effort of the system to get rid of the lead, he let it have its course; the time the diarrhœa lasted seemed to be somewhat in proportion to the length of time the lead had been used. He advances the idea that possibly leaded patients might get rid of their lead by keeping them tolerably physicked for two or three weeks.

It is not generally known that lead affects the buccal cavity pretty much like quicksilver, producing an inflammation of the tonsils, palate, and gums, and salivation; and the breath has a disagreeable smell.

He has seen lead cause an apparent amelioration of the condition of consumptive patients, which, however, did not persist. But when it was a martial affection of the whole organism, lead has cured catarrhal consumption for good.

XIII. Remedies for the Trachea.

Affections of the wind pipe, such as hoarseness, tickling cough, asthma and loss of speech, may be amenable to quicksilver or the golden sulphide of antimony; this last may suffice when the hoarseness is recent, but when it is chronic, mercury generally must follow the antimony. A young girl, 15 years old, while stirring a fire of coals got her windpipe filled of smoke, and from that time lost her speech; after waiting in vain for six weeks, being no better, she consulted Rademacher, who prescribed Hahnemann's black mercury, one grain a day. One day she feels a snap in her throat, and she recovers her voice, which was as clear and distinct as before the accident.

Rademacher never met a pure, idiopathic case of asthma; all the cases he treated were reflex affections of the lungs, of the heart, or of abdominal organs; but as the primary affection is, if not incurable, at least inveterate and hard to cure, the sympathetic asthma cannot always be removed.

Carbonic acid is probably a good anti-spasmodic in asthma. A powder made of carbonate of magnesia and tartaric acid (1 oz. of the former to 3 dr. of the latter) has been used to allay asthma; the dry powder is put on the tongue, thus setting carbonic acid free which is then inhaled.

XIII. Remedies for the Œsophagus.

There is a peculiar inflammation of the gullet, which appears in connection with gastric (bilious) fevers, and is caused by an excess of acrid bile in the alimentary canal. The patient is not aware of anything until a difficulty of deglutition suddenly appears, and he sends for the physician, who sometimes may detect the inflammation in the fauces; but the inflammation may lay deeper, and cannot be seen. This dysphagia he not seldom cured in one day with the remedy governing the prevailing epidemic of hepatic affection. When caused by an excess of acid in the stomach, magnesia removed it easily. But if the patient cannot swallow this drug, it may sometimes be necessary to let him take by means of a teaspoon a solution of borax, which gradually penetrates through the constricted gullet, and thus heals the erysipelatous inflammation so that deglutition is again possible. Then a potion of magnesia should be administered without delay.

A spasmodic constriction of the muscular fibres of the gullet is soon removed by *Belladonna.*

The stricture of the œsophagus caused by induration of the tissues is well nigh incurable. Rademacher cured two or three cases of stricture with mercury and another with iodine, but he admits that these may have been caused by the inflammation and swelling of the two small glands which lay back of the œsophagus in the region of the fifth dorsal vertebra. He quotes two ancient authors, one of whom performed an autopsy on his patient who had died of starvation: The walls of the gullet were glued together on account of the compression exerted upon that tube by those pathologically enlarged glands.

C. CEPHALIC REMEDIES.

XIV. The Eye.

Although Rademacher, like any other general practitioner, only had a limited experience in diseases of the eye, yet he gives us some useful hints.

Inflammation of the eyes seldom is a symptom of a general affection, which may be cured by saltpetre, iron or copper. It may also be (and amblyopia, amaurosis, etc., as well) a sympathetic affection caused by hyperacidity of the alimentary canal, in which case laxatives or antacids are the remedy, or it may be a reflex of a primary affection of some other organ, which organ must first be cured.

The selection of the remedy for eye diseases changes with the time, one year requiring this remedy, another year that one; during an epidemic of contagious, extremely painful ophthalmy, the water of bitter almonds was the only remedy that cured it.

Eye remedies used externally are generally employed too strong. Rademacher cured with a salve consisting of one grain of *mercurius cinereus* and two drachms of lard ophthalmias which had resisted strong mercurial salve. The same is true of the sublimate; with a solution of one grain in 16 ounces of water, inflammations of the eye may be cured which a stronger solution could not remove. A solution of 1 drachm of borax in 6 ounces of water, or one of 1 grain of acetate of zinc in 1 ounce of water are very good. Another good eye salve is one made from one drachm of lard and one or two grains of a mild silver salt, the composition of which will be given under the brain remedies.

Ethereal, aromatic oils, when allowed to evaporate under the eye, are very beneficial; the most efficacious is the oil of majoram, one drop being dropped on a piece of linen which is then held before the eye.

XV. The Nose.

Nose affections, such as loss of smell, chronic coryza, ulceration, are often reflex symptoms of an abdominal affection; cure this, and the other will disappear, too. A common cold can be cured in short time by snuffing camphor powder and taking cubic saltpetre internally.

Nose bleed, too, is often of reflex origin, and may be caused by an irregular circulation in the portal system, or by obstructions of the liver or of the spleen. The internal use of the powdered seed of carduus marianus is then the best remedy. But nosebleed may be a symptom of a martial (universal affection) in which case give the muriate of iron.

XVI. The Mouth.

Ulceration or cancer of the tongue are often caused by the sharp edges of some broken or ulcerated teeth, or by some sharp calcareous concretion on the inner side of the teeth. Filing the sharp tooth, and removing the concretion is generally sufficient to allay the inflammation, if not gone too far. In all inflammations of the tongue, especially of the edges, the physician should look for this.

For the thrush of children, borax is the best remedy, but antacids are indispensable, and must be given to the mother as well, if the child sucks; sweets are a fruitful source of hyperacidity of the stomach; hence, thrush and other disorders.

Chronic tonsillitis is often a local manifestation of a martial disease of the whole system, then iron is the best remedy. But it may be caused by hyperacidity of the stomach or bowels; then alkalies are required. Sometimes the portal system is at fault, and sulphur is the remedy. Hypertrophied tonsils can sometimes be cured with iodine salve externally and a gargling of 8 ounces of water and 16 drops of iodine.

Rademacher once cured with muriate of lime a fungus growing on the inner side of the gum of an incisor; it was very painful, and the pain spread from the jaw to the nostril of the same side. The fungus was removed by a surgeon, but returned; Rademacher then applied a solution of one part of muriate of lime in two parts of water, and the persistent use of this lotion removed the growth. Five years later the fungus had not returned.

Toothache is often the local manifestation of a general affection curable with saltpetre, and Rademacher has often cured it with large doses of this salt. It is necessary to give Glauber's salt or some other laxative at the same time, if the patient is constipated. When it is a purely local affection, it may be cured with zinc, or with tobacco spirit.

Not seldom a sound tooth is very painful, being sympathetically affected by a carious tooth in some other part of the jaw, and queer enough, the rotten tooth may be painless; by pulling out the carious tooth, the pain will disappear from the sound one. What is true of other organs is true of the teeth, viz., a pain is a very delusive indicator of the primarily affected organ.

When a body, otherwise well, is suddenly attached with an inflammation of the parotid gland, accompanied with fever, the internal use of *Natrum nitricum* (½ oz. in 24 hours), with 30 or 40 drops of tincture of iodine, and externally a salve of zinc oxide will cure it in a short time; but if the bowels are costive, give Glauber's salt or some other laxative. In chronic inflammation of the parotid gland the internal and external use of iodine is excellent.

This salve of zinc oxide externally, with some cubic saltpetre internally, when there is fever, is good to resolve the inflammation of the submaxillary glands of children.

XVII. Brain Remedies.

Tobacco.

In June, 1819, brain fevers appeared, against which Rademacher learned to use tobacco. From 1816 to 1819 gastric fevers had predominated, which were cured with alkalies and the tincture of nux vomica. In their first stage both diseases differed very little; both had severe headache, strong fever with a full, quick pulse; the tongue was slightly coated, and the color of the urine changeable. The inefficacy of the antacids and hepatics showed him that another kind of disease was at hand, against which he was impotent.

The symptoms differed according to the patients. Some had toothache as forerunner of the fever; in some cases it ended with toothache; others had buzzing in the ears, some had inflamed eyes; in a few, the fever started with violent vomiting, and a few had diarrhœa. The only characteristic symptom was a severe headache which in some patients seized the whole head, in some the posterior part of the head, and in others only the region of the cerebellum; it was constant, without remission. This fever, left to itself, presented the same symptoms as typhoid, viz., a dry tongue, debility, subsultus tendinum, diarrhœa, and sometimes delirium. Cubic saltpetre diminished the fever, but the headache remained the same.

While waiting in the pharmacy for a prescription, Rademacher's attention was called to an old herbal of Dodoneus, and opening it at random, his eye caught the description of the tobacco plant, to which old physicians attributed wonderful virtues; after reading the article, he thought that either the tobacco plant must be a remedy for the diseased brain and spine, or else the old physicians were all knaves. Being in need of a good cephalic, he decided to try it, and had the druggist prepare a tincture from the fresh leaves of the *Nicotiana rustica*, growing in his garden. He gave to some of his patients who suffered mostly of headache without fever half an ounce of the tincture in twenty-four hours; its effects were excellent, but as it acted on the bowels, and he feared an aggravation of the diarrhœa which sometimes accompanied this disease, he had the druggist distil a spirit from the tincture; this spirit of tobacco acted like a charm, removing the headache, and the diarrhœa, and with it he could not only treat, but cure the disease. But as he had found from previous experience that the cubic saltpetre allayed the fever (without, however, curing the disease), he mixed 2 drachms of cubic saltpetre, half an ounce of spirit of tobacco, and 8 ounces of water, giving the patient one spoonful every hour. The disease was sometimes cured in three or four days, but in general it took from eight to ten days, if the above mixture was administered in the first stage; but if two or more weeks had elapsed before the doctor was called in, the tobacco and saltpetre did no good; however by substituting peroxide of iron, and 10 grains of tragacanth (so that the iron would not fall so easily from the mixture), the disease could be cured as before. In some cases where Rademacher was called so late that the patients were perfectly delirious, zinc not only removed the delirium, but the whole disease. Later, Rademacher used instead of the *Spiritus nicotianæ* an *Aqua spirituosa* which has all the virtues of the spirit, and of which one-half or a full ounce can be given in twenty-four hours, without causing either vomiting or diarrhœa.

Rademacher is inclined to think that the tobacco affects specially the cerebellum and the spine, since the occipital pain was the only constant symptom of this epidemic. Future observations may elucidate this point.

Thornapple (*Stramonium*).

The above described brain fevers continued until 1821 when the spirit of tobacco began to fail to cure, and Rademacher perceived that another epidemic influence was at work. In this new disease the severe headache was not located in the occiput, but in the forehead and in the crown; it was not so persisteut, as it abated somewhat, but during its exacerbation the pain was terrible, and was sometimes accompanied with delirium which disappeared during the remission of the pain. This headache was the only certain symptom by which this disease differed from the preceding; there was no vomiting, but the diarrhœa was more frequent, and often a very troublesome cough made its appearance. The disease, left to itself, lasted very long, sheer exhaustion merely putting an end to it; in one patient it lasted from the 11th of September to the 27th of December. Cubic saltpetre instead of allaying the fever and the diarrhœa only increased this last symptom. The acetate of iron reduced the fever, at the same time stopping the diarrhœa and nosebleed which was very detrimental to the patient; but the headache remained and the disease continued its course.

To Rademacher this disease seemed to be a mixed one, viz., a martial affection combined with an idiopathic, primary brain affection. The question now was to find an organ remedy for the brain. After trying in vain the cephalic remedies of the old physicians, *Hypericum* and *Anagallis*, his thoughts were directed to *Stramonium*, which he had once used with success in a case of severe, periodic, daily headache; he now found the remedy which conquered the obstinate headache. His supposition that this was a mixed affection proved true, for *Stramonium* alone cured this disease just as little as the iron alone. But in mixing one ounce of simple tincture of acetate of iron, one ounce of gum arabic, one drachm of *Stramonium* tincture and seven ounces of water, to be taken in twenty-four hours, a spoonful every hour, he had the true remedy. The vascular irritability and the headache were speedily allayed, a steady amelioration set in, and the interminable disease was cured in a period of eight to fourteen days. In some patients the brain affection was accompanied by a very painful ophthalmy, but this also disappeared under the use of iron and *Stramonium.*

CHLORIDE OF SILVER.

This is probably the *Argentum lasureum* of Paracelsus, which he praises as a cephalic remedy. Rademacher accidentally learned to prepare it from Woyt's Treasury, an old German medical dictionary. However, he never had much occasion to use it until 1824.

The brain fevers just described continued till about the month of September of that year, and then the mixture of *Stramonium* and iron failed to act. Rademacher looked for another cephalic and found the chloride of silver to be the remedy for the new epidemic. While in the two previous epidemics the headache had been a prominent symptom, in this one it was seldom observed, but in its stead, all patients complained of dizziness. When called in early, Rademacher could at once bring the patient to convalescence; but if called late, when the typhoid stage had been reached, when delirium, sopor, subsultus tendinum, a dry tongue, diarrhœa, etc., were present, the recovery took two weeks, although silver was and remained the only remedy.

ZINC.

Of the brain remedies zinc is the one which Rademacher used the earliest and the oftenest, although he never saw an epidemic which it did cure in its first stage. It is best combined with acetic acid; the ordinary dose of the acetate is 1½ drachms, never more than 2, and sometimes even less than 1½ drachms, dissolved in 8 ounces of water, to which one ounce of gum arabic has been added. If it is employed for chronic cases, it is best to give it in the form of pills, on account of the dislike its continuous use produces.

Rademacher calls zinc the mineral opium, on account of its sedative virtues. He tried it on himself, and it made him so sleepy that he could not collect his thoughts. With it he has cured the most painful ophthalmias, severe toothache, earache, neuralgia, sciatica, and painful gout and rheumatism. Zinc cures in twenty-four hours that grave form of facial erysipelas coupled with severe fever and delirium, when the face and the scalp are covered with large blisters. This form of erysipelas, when not checked, may end in insanity, and must well be distinguished from the milder form of erysipelas, caused by some abdominal organ or by hyperacidity of the stomach or bowels, or by abnormal bile secretion.

Although zinc never cured a brain fever in its first stage, yet it proved an indispensable remedy when the headache turned into a continuous delirium, or into sopor; then the zinc not only removed the delirium or sopor, but cured the whole disease. This lasting delirium is very different from the periodic delirium, as regards therapeutics; when the last symptom prevailed, zinc only caused a temporary amelioration, while *Stramonium* (with iron) cured. It affords the physician much satisfaction to bring with zinc a raving patient to his senses within twenty-four hours sometimes. But as long as the patient has still some lucid moments during which he complains of headache, it is best to give some remedy like *Stramonium* instead of zinc, and thus prevent a relapse and a disappointment; but when the delirium becomes contant and intensified, so that the patient does not complain any more of headache, but is either stupid, as if struck with apoplexy, or else raving like a maniac, then zinc is the remedy; a calm sleep succeeds the delirium. But do not think the battle won; if allowed to sleep on after the first dose, he will awake as delirious as before; but if his nurse wakes him up to give him his medicine (zinc) every hour, until he awakes spontaneously, and acts and speaks rationally, only then is it safe to think the danger over. Even then zinc must be continued for a couple of days, but in smaller dose, or at longer intervals. It is the same when acute brain affections end in sopor; zinc is the remedy here, too, and the stupid patient awakes spontaneously when zinc has done its work; but even before that, every time that the patient is wakened up, which must be done every hour, to give him his medicine, it will be observed that the mental powers are gradually returning.

Rademacher cites an interesting case when the raving delirium was changed by zinc into deep stupor, with perfect recovery. He was called to a man who, after suffering with fever and a violent headache for four days, had suddenly become insane. A potion of 2 drachms of zinc with 1 ounce of gum arabic in 8 ounces of water, was left with his wife, with the instruction to give him a spoonful every hour. The wife, hoping to get rid of her husband whom she hated, gave him this potion in quick doses, thinking it might kill him; but, instead, he fell into a deep sleep;

the next day, when Rademacher visited him, he was still sleeping, but when wakened up the delirium was gone; the same potion was left to be administered every hour, and the next day he was free of fever, delirium and sopor, to the great chagrin of his wife.

Sympathy Between Brain and Abdominal Organs.

Brain diseases easily cause reflex abdominal affections, the stomach, the bowels, and the liver being much oftener affected than the spleen, or the pancreas, or the kidneys, although in 1831 Rademacher often saw sympathetic affections of the spleen. When the brain disease had not been preceded by any other disease, these reflex affections did not require any special remedies. But when previous abdominal diseases were sympathetically stirred up by a brain affection, the cephalic remedy was not capable to cure the brain disease in its first stage, but the latter went into the second stage, characterized by the constant delirium. Sometimes the abdominal affection was so serious that it became idiopathic, and then not zinc, but the appropriate abdominal remedy alone, could remove the whole disease.

On the other hand, most mental disorders have their cause in some abdominal affection, while the least are idiopathic brain affections. The following case may serve as illustration. A farmer became insane, on account of a bad land speculation, if the information of his friends was correct. But as his urine had a darker shade than the normal, and as bilious fevers had been prevailing, Rademacher gave him celandine, since of all hepatics this is the best to cure a disease of the liver which sympathetically affects the brain. Neither did it fail to cure in this case.

Although it is proper in mental disorders to direct the remedies to the abdominal organs when these seem clearly at fault, this does not always succeed; the abdominal remedy may bring an amelioration that is not lasting, and instead of belaboring the belly with other abdominal remedies, to the detriment of the brain disease, which in the meantime grows stronger, it is prudent to try a brain remedy, as the two following cases will show.

A young man, appointed administrator of the estate of minor children was accused, after having discharged himself of this duty, of having misappropriated some of the estate. This brought on insanity. As there existed at the same time a sympathetic abdominal affection Rademacher treated him for two weeks with hepatics, but in vain; neither the brain nor the abdominal affection got any better. He now tried the acetate of zinc, which cured him in four days of his insanity and of his sympathetic abdominal affection.

A twenty year old girl, in service with over-religious people, lost her reason, probably on account of burdening her mind with religious scruples and doubts. As she had much eructation, her tongue was coated, the urine dark, and gastric diseases were then prevailing, Rademacher gave her a mixture of tincture of nux vomica and asafœtida, thinking that her insanity was but a reflex of a hepatic disease. Two weeks after, she was apparently as rational as she had ever been. But the amelioration was only temporary, for the insanity returned, and although she was given the same remedy, she got rather worse. Rademacher thought it best to now try a brain remedy; he gave her an 8 ounce potion containing 1½ drachms of acetate of zinc and 1 ounce gum arabic, a spoonful every hour. After taking five such potions, she was cured of her insanity and of her gastric trouble. She remained sane.

In closing his chapter on brain remedies Rademacher offers the following remarks: "Probably all brain remedies (but from experience I can speak only of zinc and tobacco) can be used to advantage, not only in pathological affections of the brain and spine, but also in idiopathic affections of other organs, when these two first are in normal condition. Without writing at length upon this point, I have in the preceding pages communicated some of my experience in this regard; but I now want to remark, it is possible that the most severe and most fatal affections of the intestinal canal or of the abdominal ganglions are sometimes better removed with brain remedies than with the best tried abdominal remedies. My experience upon this subject is too imperfect to let me communicate it in abstract practical propositions, and to tell it in all the details would take too long; but I hope that the mere mention of this probably important subject will be sufficient to urge thinking physicians to further investigations."

In another place, when commenting upon the severe and painful cramps of the lower extremities, the remarkable coldness of the whole body and the terribly distorted face seen in cholera, he adds: "It seems to me probable that in this disease the brain or the spine are primarily diseased, while the intestinal canal is only sympathetically affected." It may, therefore, not be out of place to bring here a few cases of cholera which he cured.

At the end of the summer of 1834 Rademacher was called to a sixty year old mechanic who had been attacked with cholera in the morning. He saw him at noon. The patient complained of dizziness, had a disagreeable sensation in the abdomen, especially at the epigastrium; he vomited without effort a watery stuff, which contained no bile, and had copious, watery stools, devoid of feces, mucus or blood. The most troublesome symptom he complained of was the painful cramps in the calfs of the legs; the pulse was small, a little accelerated, but not irregular, the tongue and the skin were cold, and his mind a little bit cloudy, just as is often the case at the beginning of brain fever. The prescription was a mixturs of 1 ounce of distilled water of tobacco, with 2 drachms of acetate of soda, dissolved in 8 ounces of water with some gum arabic a spoonful every hour. Toward evening the doctor visited him, and found that the vomiting had ceased, the first spoonful of the remedy had been retained; the cramps were considerably lessened, and the patient had had only a couple of watery stools devoid of feces. The coldness of the skin and of the tongue was gone, and the temperature was normal; but the dizziness was unchanged. The next morning the condition was much better. The patient had had a copious normal passage, after which the nauseous sensation had left the epigastrium; the urine was a little darker than the normal; the dizziness was less, and the night had not been passed without some little sleep. The medicine was continued, and on the morning of the third day the dizziness was entirely gone, the patient had had a good sleep and was well.

Rademacher remarks, after citing two similar cases:

"Whether you call the disease dysentery, brain fever or cholera, it is all the same. That is a mere formality, and has nothing to do with its real nature and its cure. The main thing is and remains to find the organ that is primarily affected, and to cure it. In this case the organ primarily affected was the brain, not the belly."

"So long as I have practiced, I never learned to know a remedy which had such a prompt, beneficial, almost magical effect, as that mixture. In the first case (not cited here) I gave the volatile spirit of tobacco as a brain remedy, because I could not possibly consider as idiopathic intestinal affection the tumultuous intestinal symptoms, and much less so the extraordinary painful cramps of the feet, which caused a strong, stout hearted man to continually cry for help, but I had necessarily to consider these as reflex symptoms of the primarily affected brain. I merely added the acetate of soda to first quiet down the stomach; for how could the volatile spirit of tobacco exert its curative effects upon the brain or the spine, if it was immediately thrown up? But although I supposed that this mixture had the desired effect, I was far from expecting such a truly magical one."

"I know of no dead sure remedy against any nosological form, cholera not excepted. But taking it for granted that the abdominal, nervous and muscular disorders which represent the disease, cholera, are the reflex of an idiopathic brain disease, does it follow from this supposition that the idiopathic brain affection shall forever be cured by the volatile spirit of tobacco, now as well as in three or four or ten years? This deduction is not to be granted. For I have treated brain fevers, which I had to cure with *Stramonium*, and others which I had to cure with silver; who will warrant me that sooner or later the brain affection, from which the cholera, as a disease form, depends, will not sometime require those remedies? Yea, who will warrant me that it will not be of such nature that I may know of no remedy for it?"

The proposition laid down by Rademacher in the preceding pages that it may be possible that the most severe and most fatal affections of the intestinal canal or of the abdominal ganglions are sometimes better removed with brain remedies than with the best tried abdominal remedies, has, no doubt, been written in regard to dysentery and cholera, which he considers as brain diseases, being caused, he thinks, by a constriction of the muscular fibres of the gut (as evidenced by the watery discharges, devoid of feces) and accompanied (the cholera at least) by cramps in the calves and by dizziness; we have seen that in the few cases of Asiatic cholera, his tried brain remedy, tobacco (with acetate of soda as a stomach sedative) was capable of overcoming this terrible disease. As Rademacher did not care to explain himself at great length upon this point, it was thought best to insert here some of the experience he gained in treating cholera, and dysentery. However, he must not be understood as considering dysentery and cholera as one and the same disease, for in the first named disease he notices the absence of coldness, cramps and distorted features which are common to cholera.

D. REMEDIES FOR EXTERNAL ORGANS.

These organs are the skin, the muscles, the ligaments, the bones, the glands, the nerves and the blood-vessels. Rademacher knew very few remedies for these organs.

XVIII. Skin Remedies.

Copper is a good remedy for some cutaneous diseases, as has been seen. Carbonate of copper made into a salve with wax removes warts and other vegetations of this kind. Rademacher used it often to hasten the suppuration of enlarged glands or of hard tumors.

The internal use of lime water (mixed with milk) has often cured milk crust. Sometimes he succeeded with a solution of borax externally.

The external use of sublimate is excellent against the itch; one-half a drachm of Sublimate and one-half a drachm of salmiac are dissolved in one pound of water, and the parts affected are washed once every other day, and allowed to dry; the first and second lotions promote the full and complete eruption of the itch pustules, while the third lotion cures it, and dries it up.

For young children and for such patients who have a very tender skin, the external use of dry sulphur, rubbed on the inside of the shirt and of the stockings, or sulphur wrapped in a piece of muslin proved very beneficial, and was sufficient to cure the itch, or bad cases of tetters (herpes). The physician must be cautious in using a solution of sublimate, as it is apt to aggravate inflammations of external parts, if used too freely, while a weak solution used at long intervals is generally very beneficial.

Dry, aromatic plants, marjoram especially, are very useful, when boiled in wine and laid on contusions; they may be used dry, with or without wrapping of cheese cloth.

A salve made of quicksilver and lead (℞ Mercurii præcipitati albi ℈i, Plumbi carbonici, axungiæ porci āā ℥ ½. M.) has in his hands often proved an excellent remedy against obstinate tetters, which had resisted the external use of sublimate, although the reverse has proved true, too.

With the acetate of zinc he has removed venereal chancres much better than with mercury, using one scruple for one ounce of water.

Table salt, too, has proved a good remedy for herpes; once he saw a tetter on the palm of a gentleman cured with the external use of a saturated solution of salt; this affection had resisted the application of a mercurial salve, as well as that of chloride of lime.

The muriate of lime is an excellent remedy for furuncles or boils, not only curing them when they are fully developed, but preventing their development when they are coming out. This remedy is applied externally, one ounce being dissolved in two pounds of water, and a wad of cotton soaked in it laid on the swelling or on the ulcer. With this simple remedy he cured some very serious and painful cases.

XIX. Muscle Remedies.

It is pretty hard to find muscle remedies proper, because the muscles are in close sympathy with almost all organs. They are in close relation with the kidneys, for instance; therefore, the acute wandering rheumatism as well as the chronic local rheumatism are not seldom idiopathic renal affections, and are often radically and speedily cured with cochineal. The muscles stand in close connection with the brain and the spine, hence brain remedies, such as tobacco and zinc, have many times cured muscular affections. Then again rheumatism and gout may be a universal affection, curable with one of the three universal remedies.

Arnica montana is very likely a muscle remedy proper; with an infusion of the flowers Rademacher has cured local rheumatism, characterized by fixed pains; for instance, a man, who after sweating, had exposed his nape and occiput to a cold winter wind was afflicted with a rheumatism of those parts; the affection, which had resisted many so-called antirheumatics, was cured in three days by drinking every evening three cups of a warm infusion of ten grains of arnica flowers. In another patient, also cured by arnica, the pain occupied the left frontal eminence and the left eye, and appeared in paroxysms, with marked remissions.

Ash leaves (*folia fraxini*) have proved very beneficial in arthritic pains, in podagra, and in rheumatism of the external parts of the head; one ounce of the leaves are steeped half an hour in hot water, and the infusion is drunk during the day.

Digitalis salve (Unguent ceræ ℥i, Extr. digitalis ʒii) rubbed on inflamed joints or limbs in rheumatism, or even in sciatica, wonderfully allays the pains in a very short time. It is excellent, too, for inflamed glands, of the armpit, for instance, or for gathered breasts, or for the indurated parotid gland; this salve not only assuages the pain, but dissipates the tumor as well.

Iodine salve, too, is sometimes very beneficial for painful affections of the muscles. Rademacher cites the following interesting case: A laborer injured the index of the right hand with a nail; the wound was insignificant, but the patient became insane. Rademacher, called in, brought him to his senses by means of the acetate of zinc, but the hand remained swollen and hard as a board, without showing any redness or other signs of inflammation. The hand was now gently rubbed for half an hour with iodine salve, morning and evening; after using the salve twice, the swelling diminished considerably, and the fingers could be moved. The amelioration continued from day to day, and in ten days the hand was entirely cured.

Nux vomica is another remedy which used externally has proved very serviceable in local, painful rheumatism, equal parts of nux vomica tincture and of spirits of soap being mixed and rubbed on the painful limb for half an hour twice a day. This remedy is not recommended against the wandering acute rheumatism, but only in local affections.

Involuntary muscular motions, or chorea, may be caused by worms or by disorders of the menstruation. Generally the feet are affected first, and the disorder gradually spreads to other groups of muscles. Rademacher found Glauber's salt the best remedy for this affection, when the patients are habitually costive. Two ounces of sulphate of soda are dissolved in two pounds of water, and the patient is directed to take a cup or a glassful every hour or two, until the bowels are moved three or four times daily; the quantity of salt is diminished from time to time, just enough being given to have three or four passages in a day. A visible amelioration is soon perceptible, generally in two weeks; by continuing this simple remedy the disease is entirely removed.

Rademacher once was called in consultation to a case of chorea which a learned physician had been unable to cure, in spite of his knowledge. Well knowing the disposition of his confrere, he avoided mentioning any new remedy, but rather proposed omitting all drugs for two weeks, and, turning to the parents of the patient, advised them to give the girl enough Glauber's salt, dissolved in water, to move her bowels three or four times a day, for since she was of a costive habit, and was not to receive any drugs, it would not do to let her be constipated for a fortnight. The wise confrere gave his consent with a sarcastic smile, as if he thought that Rademacher was merely hiding his ignorance and helplessness. In two weeks the chorea was so much better that nobody thought of using any other remedy than the Glauber's salt solution which finished the cure.

It seems as if the sulphate of soda was beneficial in those cases only where the bowels are costive. In the case of a young woman whose bowels were regular the salt accomplished nothing; artemisia powder, a heaped teaspoon, five times a day, diminished the involuntary muscular motion, but the amelioration stopped after a week; then the acetate of zinc was tried, and this proved the true remedy, although the cure took a long time, on account of the dislike of the patient to the taste of the zinc.

A most remarkable case of nervous or muscular disorder, cured with Glauber's salt, is worth being translated in its most important details: One afternoon, in 1840, Rademacher was invited by a stranger to visit his daughter, who, he said, had a strange attack every afternoon. The patient was a pretty maiden who, according to external appearance, did not appear sick in the least. She had been treated by two experienced physicians, one of whom had prescribed quinine, on account of the periodicity of the disease, without any success however. While Rademacher was reading the prescriptions used in her case, the attack came on her; she had been sitting on a chair by the window, but her father took her and laid her on the bed, and the doctor had the occasion to witness the strange spectacle of the double form of a disease. The left side of her body was seized with a tetanic spasm, the arm stretched close to the body and so stiff that it was impossible to move it in the least. The right side, on the contrary, was in a convulsive, trembling condition, and the maiden was gesticulating with the arm of that side, making the same involuntary motions as those afflicted with chorea. She was given Glauber's salt, with the result that some twelve days later the father sent word that she was much better; but as the salt was purging her rather freely, he wanted to know whether it was to be discontinued. Rademacher sent him word to keep up its use, but in smaller doses, and about one month later he received word that the girl was entirely healed.

LAST WORD OF RADEMACHER TO THE READER.

"My old master Hufeland told me to prove all things, and to choose the best. * * * I have called your attention to a foundation of the medical art (the curative action of the drugs) which has been misjudged or overlooked, and believe thereby to have accomplished something useful, if not worthy of thanks. Whatever choice you may make after mature examination is your business, not mine. My position in life is not such as could influence your reason. I am as free as any one in Germany, and being under no obligations except those of good morals and the laws of the land, no social conditions compel me to play the trickster as physician or as writer. Finally, being neither a learned man, nor a philosopher, neither a university professor nor a titled man, but merely a plain medical practitioner, living in a little town, to help townsmen and farmers, and having shown myself to you without any varnish, but as nature made me, without any disposition to be a sophist, your reason, if it is free of the trammels of the time, has the most perfect freedom to prove all things and to select the best."

INDEX